Retire to GREAT FRIENDSHIPS

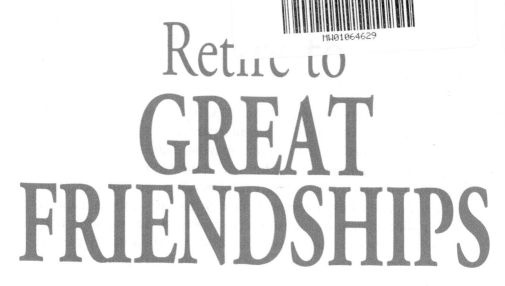

How to grow your network of fun and support

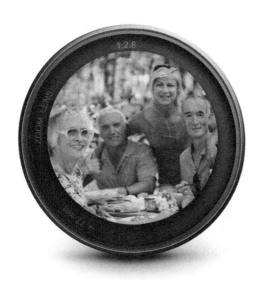

Ed Zinkiewicz

Retire to Great Friendships: How to grow your network of fun and support

ISBN (Perfectbound): 978-0-9886622-6-1
ISBN (e-Book): 978-0-9886622-7-8

Cover design and interior layout by Bookcovers.com

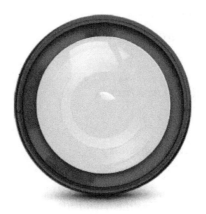

Table of Contents

Part 1: Oops! Where did they all go?

Part 2: So, now what?

For You and Footnotes

A website has been created for this book. You can find it at:

www.retireto.info/friendships/bookresources/

In general, the site has two parts:

For You: This part contains additional material you will find helpful in growing your network of fun and support. Most chapters have references at the end that explain material on the site relevant to the chapter. On the website, items are noted by chapter in the For You section.

Footnotes: All of the footnotes from this book are also on the webpage listed above. Some of the footnotes contain web links, which are active there. Just click on them and go directly to the referenced page. In the print version of this book all the web links are shortened. They are limited to their simple home page URL, which makes them easier to type into your browser.

For other resources to help you make your retirement the best of your life, go to retire-to.com.

Bonuses

You may have purchased this book at a brick and mortar or an online bookstore. As a result, you may not have known about the bonuses available to you for purchasing the book.

Don't miss out on these freebies. Just send an email to friendships@retire-to.com; tell me where you bought the book, if you got this book as a gift and whether you have a paper or electronic version. We'll do the rest.

We'll send you:

Listen Now or Pay Later. This is an audio of "Commandment Number 3" in Drs. Brad and Ted Klontzs' wonderful resource entitled, *The Ten Commandments for Extraordinary Relationships* (copyright © 2006 Klontz Kahler, LLC).

I agree with the promotional summary: This CD "reviews ten relationship principles that are essential to making the most of intimate relationships. If relationships did come with an instructional manual, this would be it!" Number 3 was a perfect fit as a bonus for this book because it goes into more detail about how to listen actively.

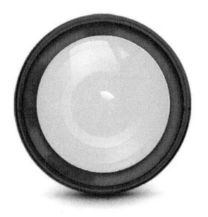

Part 1

Oops! Where did they all go?

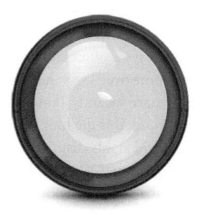

Introduction

R etirement can be a lonely place. It doesn't have to be.
I've spent a great deal of time with people in nursing homes. For ten years, I visited folks there from my church. For them, the point had come at which they could no longer care for themselves at home and they had to make the move. Every month as we visited, one complaint consistently rose to the surface: loneliness.

Close family was gone. Few friends were left, and the ones remaining could no longer travel to see them. Too frequently, the daily obituaries brought sad news. Mail was scarce and visitors scarcer. Infrequent social contact heightened their isolation.

I also regularly play music in nursing homes. In these situations, I don't connect a great deal with individuals, but I am able to stand back and observe the bigger picture. Sad as the complaints of loneliness were when I visited friends from church, what I have witnessed at the nurses' station, in the rooms, and in the hallways is often sadder. People call out for me—a stranger—to come over, to spend a minute with them, to listen. Others only stare vacantly. Loneliness is a pallor that drapes faces like a shroud. It is the look of abandonment.

These experiences and sights disturb me. Is that what my life will bring? Will I be alone? Will I be lonely?

You may have felt the same gnawing anxiety. Perhaps the anxiety is evident in the comments of a parent you cannot visit frequently or in the despair of a friend who has lost a loved one. Have you watched the eyes? Heard the lament in the voice?

Good grief, Ed. What does that have to do with retirement?

Here's something you may not expect: You pop out of the job into the bright blue of the western sky headed for the great reward you deserve—retirement! You've so looked forward to it. But in the days, weeks, and months following the retirement party, you look around and realize you've lost friends along the way.

When you comprehend what has happened, the discovery is a retirement surprise—something you didn't anticipate! Think of a surprise as a hand grenade. Grenades explode and blow up stuff!

- Bam. Will I be alone?
- Boom. Will I feel lonely?
- Yuck. Have I become one of those people in the nursing home?

Ed, I didn't ask for that! I just wanted to have a great retirement. Whose bright idea was it to bring that up? And what do you mean I've lost all my friends from work?

Of course, not everybody loses all their friends when they leave work behind. If you haven't, then good for you. But, this book is still for you! Look at the tips I've put together for keeping some of those friends near and dear—and for creating new friendships.

Then too, your experience with nursing homes may not have been as dramatic as mine. If not, I'm glad for that. Cast your net wide and look closely: Do you have friends or family members nearing the time for a move to a nursing facility? Extend your vision for their circumstance just a little ways into the future. What will happen to their circle of friends?

For those of you who are wondering what retirement may bring, read on. You cannot know what the future holds, but you will find it helpful to see how you can grow and strengthen your network of relationships. Great friendships make life interesting and enjoyable! And great friends will proof your life against the loneliness that will certainly ensue without them.

Friendships are so important. Whether you've lost friends from work, have managed to keep them so far, or don't particularly worry about the long haul as I might, scientific studies now prove multiple reasons to hang on to your friends. Having friends is vital for your well-being!

This book tackles four topics:

- What retirement might bring
- What makes friendship so important
- How to revitalize your friend network
- How to evaluate yourself as a friend

I want you to find happiness, wellness, and meaning, to feel alive and not abandoned. My wife, Crys, and I founded Retirement-U, and we lead workshops that help prepare individuals for that major life-transition called retirement. We highlight these key elements because they are important for making this time of life the best. It is our passion that you find your retirement a great place to be.

Friendship is absolutely critical to happiness, as well as a positive influence in taking care of yourself and finding meaning and purpose. So, please join me in the discovery of why friendship matters and how you can grow your network of fun and support.

I can't promise that you will never be alone or feel some loneliness. I can promise that, if you follow the steps I've outlined here, you can start today to build strong, enduring, supportive friendships—and have fun along the way.

This path is right because it is positive, moving upward toward a meaningful goal instead of downward in a spiral toward loneliness. It is a path you can take.

Why wait? Read on. You can do this!

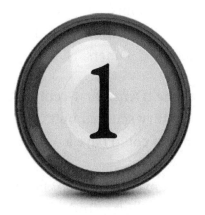

How Did I Get to Be Alone?

"What was the ref thinking?"
"Did you hear what happened?"
"How is your mom doing?"
"Are you feeling better?"
"Just how are we going to fix the project?"
"Want to see the new movie?"

When you retire, you lose...

Talking, laughing, caring—the stuff water coolers are made for! These snippets of conversations, fueled by a few chance moments or well-earned breaks happen daily at thousands of water coolers all over the United States. And not just water coolers—

Lunch rooms.   Washrooms.   Coffee nooks.
   Locker rooms.   Break rooms.   Food-vendor trucks.
      Laboratories.   Diners.   Cubbies.

These places are the twenty-first-century equivalent of the early nineteenth-century scuttled butt[1], the place on a naval vessel where shipmates could have a quiet conversation away from the officer.

Our workplace conversations go far beyond what we know today as "scuttlebutt." Today's conversations show concern, follow shared interests, evoke passionate opinion, demonstrate caring, and elicit support. The conversations are as varied in purpose as the people who gather to converse.

And these conversations are not limited to the office. These conversations are for white-collar and blue-collar workers, for dockhands and farmhands, for skilled laborers and scientists, for doctors and lawyers alike. These are *your* conversations, the stuff of life at the workplace.

The water cooler disappears

Along with it go all these conversations and most, if not all, of those people, which means less camaraderie in your life and, when you need them most, fewer humorous moments and fewer sympathetic listeners.

And if that weren't bad enough, we tend to fill these empty moments with things less vital: the remote and the mouse. Gone are personal involvement and interaction.

Being entertained at home by the TV is good, but it's not the same as creating your own hilarious moment with friends. Hearing someone else's comments at the library "author's

---

1 A cask (butt) of water with a hole, which scuttled the cask for other uses, but allowed sailors access to drinking water and a place to hang out for a few minutes and exchange pleasantries and rumors (scuttlebutt).

night" may be stimulating, but it's not in the same league as having to defend your own ideas with folks who know how to punch your hot buttons—and who still like you when all is said and done.

Of course, the workplace is not just a place to chat; it is also a place to work. Real people come together and collaborate to make something happen. You and your coworkers deliver a service, produce a product, generate ideas, or plan for all manner of campaigns.

And you do these essential tasks together. Sometimes you even cooperate in a way that has a multiplier effect on what would otherwise be individual efforts. Individuals derive a larger sense of purpose from efforts achieved together. Coaches have told us that for centuries.

We work better as a team. Together the team can win. But, as any good coach would admit, we can't belittle good teamwork by limiting it to cheering, "Rah rah, go team!" A team is a place where we

- Learn trust and practice respect
- Engage in constructive problem solving
- Undertake mutual support
- Watch commitment in action
- Experience success
- Pull ourselves up from "failure" and begin again

Work is the place where we fight dragons together! Fire breathers! It is often challenging, sometimes risky. The tasks may strain our abilities and yet encourage new efforts. Friends are not just acquaintances, but foxhole buddies.

Facing tough challenges together creates a bond. Retirement breaks those bonds. Your life has less trust, less satisfaction from finding solutions, less support. You experience a lowered level of achievement, and you miss the encouragement needed to begin again despite a "failure."

Teamwork disappears

The work you did together no longer exists for you. Your team is gone.

The transition from being a part of a team to not a part of the team strikes at the very core of the brain where autonomic responses reside. Your teammates, your coworkers are your tribe. As humans we've lived more generations as tribesmen than as city slickers. In early times, being part of the tribe was a matter of survival. If you had a tribe, you survived. If you lost your tribe, you died.

Life is tough out there. Our brains have built-in response mechanisms that can do extremely uncivilized things when survival is threatened. The brain reacts automatically. When threatened with loss of tribe, we feel stress. The autonomic responses to stress are fight, flight, and freeze. Push a button; the bell rings. It is just that simple.

Is it any wonder, then, that some people withdraw socially at retirement? These people replace human interaction with isolated and isolating defaults: TV remote and computer mouse. Retired women over 65 watch an hour more of TV per day (3.74) than the average American. Retired men watch an hour more than that (4.73)! People over 75 watch more TV than any other group.[2] These folks have replaced half of the hours previously devoted to work with watching TV.

Unfortunately, when you leave the tribe, your need to connect with others cannot be adequately met with simulated conversation on the TV. No matter what is said on the

---

2 "What Retirees Do All Day," by Emily Brandon, *US News and World Report*, July 2, 2012.

screen, *you* are not doing the talking. You can't even practice your active listening skills—no one is on the other end to hear your feedback. You are not involved with people by watching TV.

A word about social networks

While social networks such as Facebook can help you keep in touch, these networks don't replace touching.[3] You are not there in person. You can't watch body language or note facial expressions. You can't hear inflections that give you clues to the meaning behind the words.

Don't get me wrong. I love Facebook. With distant relatives or friends, Facebook allows more contact than I otherwise would have.

More on Facebook

PROS

Connect: Long-distance friends can be closer.

Share the fun: You make a chess move. Your friend makes a move. You don't have to be playing at the same time of day!

Fit your schedule: You don't have to be on Facebook at a particular time.

Use it wherever: Have time at lunch? Are you waiting in line to pick up grandkids? No problem.

CONS

No privacy: Ask some young adults if they've ever posted something on Facebook that they wouldn't want their boss—current or potential—to see. Any kind of at-risk behavior will be discovered. Orwell was right— Big Brother is watching. In fact, we help him out by posting our own incriminating evidence!

Well, I don't need that job anyway; I'm retired!

Maybe so. But what about a prospective life mate? retirement community? landlord?

---

3 I'm not picking on Facebook. It happens to be the service most people, including me, spend their time with if they use social networks at all, according to 2011 data from socialnomics.net. I believe my comments are true for any of the dozens of similar services, as well.

Facebook is also fun. We can share challenges, comment on issues, work on projects, play games. We're part of a community, which is interacting. I show pictures of my grandkid and my friends show theirs.

I realize, however, that with that medium I can share only a portion of my life. And games with a remote buddy cannot replace a live connection. Yes, you can interact with others by playing a game on the computer. But, how much planning is involved? Do you work with your team to decide the best options?

If your buddy is a few thousand miles away, it can be a way to share a favorite pastime. But where is the personal interaction if you make your Scrabble move at midnight and your friend adds tiles at 2 P.M.?

Yikes, work happens every day!

The workplace is also not just the workplace. The workplace is an automatic means of making acquaintance. On one hand, a group of you may be thrown together on the tenth floor to finish the framing of a new set of offices. Or you might be one of the folks who meet in one of those offices to set corporate direction for the company. In the process you find companions.

You go to lunch. You ride the elevator together. You commute with others from work. You play on the same bowling league or meet for a regular lunchtime pinochle group. You play the games together at the yearly Christmas party. You clap in recognition of the most recent five-year pin recipients. You say "Hi" to each other when you come in and "Bye" when you leave.

And you do that every day!

Work is like a fishbowl. For eight hours a day you are thrust into the same environment. You have a lot in common and a place to share it.

When you retire, the fellowship environment disappears.

Retirement means you have no regular place to go every day. People don't greet you when you arrive or say goodbye when you leave. The people you could count on to miss you if you didn't show up may actually miss you, but cannot show care to you on a daily basis. The lunchroom disappears. The water cooler is broken.

In fact, if work is a fishbowl, retirement is like smashing it with a hammer. For you, the retiree, the fish are gone; the "school" and all the activity you did together are gone; the bowl is gone. You can be isolated. You can be lonely. When you retire, you can face a life less involved, less interesting, and less meaningful.

And then it gets worse

While you were working for a living, did you have a lot of time to develop friendships outside of work? Hey, "Get a life" is a TV gag. It doesn't really mean anything in the real world where most folks are doing two people's jobs, commuting endlessly, and missing sleep. In some of the jobs I have had, I did not have time to figure out how to "get a life." I was too busy. Many people are in the same boat with just not a lot of time available outside of work.

Besides, you have friends at work. Right? When you work, you don't perceive the need to take the extra effort to make more friends. The friendship ticket has been punched. You have buddies to do things with and even fewer hours to create more friends because you're spending time with the buddies you have already.

You know what that means? When you retire, there may not be a lot of friends hanging around waiting for you to have extra time.

My wife has a friend, Emma, who visits every year. Crys and Emma have been friends for more than 60 years, which is very unusual. How many friends have you had since childhood? I only vaguely recollect the names of kids I played with growing up, and I certainly would not recognize them if I met them on the street now. I received some pictures of a recent high school reunion, and except for the one man with a nametag, I could not identify any of the people.

What happens to your friends?

- **People move**. Jobs, school, and family are all strong incentives to relocate. Particularly at retirement time, it is not uncommon for people to move to be near grandchildren or aging parents.
- **People find new interests.** Things that once drew you together no longer do so.
- **People die**.

And one other common reason you lose friends: *You* may move away! How many people do you know who have relocated after retirement?

Dr. Irene S. Levine, the author of *Best Friends Forever: Surviving a Breakup with Your Best Friend*, surveyed more than 1,500 women between the ages of 17 and 70. She says:

> *I learned that most friendships, even very good ones, don't last forever. Yet women are raised to believe the romanticized notion of BFF (best friends forever), a myth that is reinforced by the media and our mothers.*[4]

4 "Why Friendships Are So Important," by Sheryl Kraft. She quotes Dr. Levine in this article. http://www.healthywomen.org/content/blog-entry/why-friendships-are-so-important

You realize what this means? If you don't *do something* to keep them, then at retirement with leaving the workplace, a dearth of other acquaintances, and attrition, you will have few, if any, friends.

For You

To get you going on the right track, I've included a fishbowl inventory for you. Take a look now:

www.retireto.info/friendships/bookresources/

The inventory provides a convenient way to help you keep in touch with friends from work. Just because you left doesn't necessarily mean you have nothing to share with the folks back there. You know—the ones on the inside!

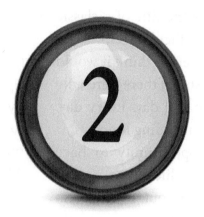

How Important Is Friendship?

Can't live without friends (literally)

Would *not* having friends be so bad? Would you miss friends and all the trimmings?

I have a friend who insists that he could live in a cave. Give him a book, and he would be a happy camper. I could not do that. While I love to read, I would not fare well with just books for company.

And while I love my wife dearly and spend a lot of time with her already, I don't think I could spend my every waking moment with just her for company. Wouldn't that level of intensity drive some retirement relationships off the rails?

For better or for worse, but not for lunch.[5]

---

5   On one website Abigail Thomas is credited with this quote. Then there is Sara Yogev's book entitled *A Couple's Guide to Happy Retirement: For Better or for Worse...But Not for Lunch*, Copyright © 2001, 2013 by Sara Yogev. Familius LLC. The quote seems ubiquitous.

This phrase is the title of a classic book about the difficulty couples can face after retirement. I think it would strain a relationship if there were only one relationship. All day. Every day. For every meal, including lunch.

I value the opportunity to have more people in my life.

So, if doing without won't work, and doing with only one won't work, how many relationships do we need? Why are they important?

Meaningful in a variety of ways

If you are like most people, you've had friends. Your experiences with them have formed your understanding of friendship. You did not start out knowing how to have a friend and be a friend. It took time and effort.

In your earliest years, friends were the kids you played beside. Childhood development experts call that parallel play; you were perfectly happy just being with someone. As you grew into actually playing together, different skills emerged, like negotiating, prioritizing, and cooperation. Meanwhile, a transformation took place. You learned to value your companions. You gained dialog skills. You began to share. And, as the fun grew, you added laughter.

What Is a Friend?

The discussion of friendship is as old as philosophy and religion and is touted by one famous person after another:

- **Plato**: Friends have all things in common. (Plato's Dialogues)
- **Aristotle**: What is a friend? A single soul dwelling in two bodies. (Aristotle's Diogenes Laertius, Lives of Eminent Philosophers)
- **Jesus**: Greater love has no one than this, that someone lay down his life for his friends. (John 15:13, ESV)
- **Thomas Aquinas**: There is nothing on earth to be prized more than true friendship.
- **Walter Winchell**: A real friend is one who walks in when the rest of the world walks out.
- **Muhammad Ali**: If you haven't learned the meaning of friendship, you really haven't learned anything.
- **Henry Ford**: My best friend is the one who brings out the best in me.

And while friends stand with you during fun times, they are also there when you need support. They may not be able to do anything about a situation, but sharing it makes it easier to get through. A good friend is also one you are willing to help.

You find fault with your friends and they with you. You grow with them, teach them, and learn from them. You listen to a friend and have no fear of spouting off. Because of a good friend, you are more than you might have been.

Friends don't need to fix each other. You can be yourself with a friend; you don't have to be perfect. And, they don't have to be on their best behavior around you, either.

You can achieve more because of friendship. **Motivation** and **encouragement** among friends can help you do that 5K run or lose those five pounds. To me, nothing says motivation like fun, and having a friend along is just more fun! The good-health gurus Doctors Oz and Roizen offer lots of reasons that, in addition to being fun, friendship increases longevity. They summarize the findings this way:

Make two friends and call me in the morning.[6]

In addition to motivation, a friend can provide **support**. A friend on the other end of a phone line can keep us from taking that next drink or smoking that next cigarette. A listening friend can shortstop stress, anger, fear, and depression.

Friends can also help us be **accountable**. I recently visited a local Rotary club, which gave me an interesting example. They use the buddy system to keep track of members. The buddy system has a primary goal: Help each other make the meetings.

The method they use is simple. During the meeting, if somebody is not present, they ask the buddy what's

---

6 "Friendships: A Surprising Key to Longevity," by Mehmet C. Oz, M.D. and Michael F. Roizen, M.D. 1/10/11, Realage.com

happening. This checking up is not pejorative; it is out of concern. "Is Alice OK?" or "John's really going to be tied up because his wife is in the hospital. They could use some help doing…."

I understand that other clubs pair a member who knows the ropes with a novice. That way you get a double whammy—the newbie can learn "how we do things around here," as well as how important he or she is to the group as a whole.

The buddy system is not just about attendance. It works the other way around as well. Attendance is the excuse to reach out. Attendance is about buddies: "We want you with us. We care."

For each of us, the importance of friendship is measured by what our friends mean to us. But friendship is not just about what we can deliver to each other. It is about **acceptance**, about allowing each other to be at ease, about valuing and being valued. Friends take joy from your relationship and make joy for you in turn.

Think about how many people use the Web to find "that perfect mate." Over four million people visited four of the top match-making websites

More Than Enough?

A friend by your side during illness is a special gift. Yet, here we have a strange anomaly. Too many friends can be a problem to caregivers.

The caregivers cannot afford to be overwhelmed with well-meaning requests for information or offers of service. We dare not disregard or belittle these concerns from friends. We could *organize* them, however, so that the caregiver can concentrate on giving care.

One method of doing that is through information-sharing websites such as Caring Bridge (caringbridge.org) or Meal Train (mealtrain.com). These websites offer a central place to provide status reports or organize help for meals, rides, pet care and the like. Caregivers have a "hub" where they can post information and ask for help. Friends and family have a means to provide services that will help and not get in the way.

(zoosk.com, Matchmaker.com, chemistry.com, and perfectmatch.com) during a single month in 2011.

Please note: I did not say how many people were happy with the services. I am saying that the interest shown in the services is a measure of the importance a "perfect match" has to its audience. (Numbers were not available for Match.com, eHarmony.com, and eLove.com. Estimates suggest over 11 million people visited those sites that same month, but I could not get authoritative numbers. Four million was sufficient to make the point.)

Friendship is also about being there through the rough patches. We've already spoken about accountability and support. But, being there is also needed during illness or last days of life.

Granted, much of the information provided so far is anecdotal or the experience of a few people. But there is more!

Friendship benefits can be measured

Growing scientific evidence suggests friendship can change your life for the better, improving

- How long you live
- How happy you are
- How healthy you are
- How well you recover from illness
- How well you cope with stress
- How well you resist mental health problems

In short, friendship can improve your well-being and give you hope.

Live longer

Friendships help you live longer. In the book, *The New Retirement,* author Jan Cullinane cites research showing that socially active people live longer. It is not hard to find medical journal summaries that make the same claim for populations all over the world. For example,

- *Survival time may be enhanced by strong social networks.*[7]
- *Across 148 studies (308,849 participants), [there was] a 50% increased likelihood of survival for participants with stronger social relationships. This finding remained consistent across age, sex, initial health status, cause of death, and follow-up period.*[8]

The same Public Library of Science (PLOS) study also compares lack of friendship to other causes of death:

The influence of social relationships on the risk of death are comparable with… smoking and alcohol consumption and exceed the influence of… physical activity and obesity.

Be happier

Friendships help you be happier. A 2005 study reported in the *Journal of Neurophysiology* showed that brain chemistry was activated in early stages of romantic love. It also reported a difference between this chemistry, associated with reward, desire, addiction, and euphoria, and the chemistry associated with purely physical attraction. (We're sorry to say that Iris Tse did not report whether this same chemistry was involved at later stages of romantic love.)[9]

---

7 *The Journal of Epidemiology and Community Health,* Research by Giles, Glonek, Luszcz, Andrews, November 23, 2004
8 *PLOS Medicine,* published by the Public Library of Science in 2010
9 Iris Tse report, myhealthnewsdaily.com, February 10, 2011

Fight illness

Friendships help you fight illness. *The New York Times* reported a 2006 study of approximately 3,000 nurses with breast cancer:

> *Women without close friends were four times as likely to die from the disease as women with ten or more friends. And notably, proximity and the amount of contact with a friend were not associated with survival. Just having friends was protective.*[10]

A six-year study of 700 Swedish men showed those with friends were less likely to have heart attacks.[11]

Addiction recovery programs from all corners consider friendship and learning how to make friends who are not addicted themselves as key to patient long-term recovery. You can check out the programs at Hazelden in Minnesota, Illinois, Florida, and other states (hazelden.org); Friendship House in California (friendshiphouses.org); and 202 Friendship House in Tennessee (202friendshiphouse.org) among others.

Reduce stress

Friendships help you reduce stress. Researchers from the Department of Comparative Human Development at the University of Chicago found that folks in committed relationships demonstrated less stress than single folks.[12]

Avoid mental health problems

Friendships help you avoid mental health problems. A 2002 review in the *American Journal of Sociology* relates that

10 *The New York Times* reported (April 20, 2009 by Tara Parker-Pope) a study published in *The Journal of Clinical Oncology*, March 1, 2006
11 *Psychosomatic Medicine*, Vol. 55, Issue 1, 1993
12 Kia Bryan report, fyiliving.com, Nov. 29, 2010

"single men and women have comparatively higher levels of depression, anxiety, mood disorders, adjustment problems, suicidal behavior, and other forms of psychological distress" than those people in relationships.[13]

The common thread in these studies? The people who were surviving and thriving were in

- "...a stronger social relationship..."
- "...the early stages of romantic love..."
- "...committed relationships..."

Also, the number of friends made a difference. In other words, these reports point to a need for quantity *and* quality, a robust social network. Which leads us to questions addressed in the following chapters: How many friends do you need? What skills do you need? And how do you go about building a strong network of friends?

For You

Enough with the research already. Let's hear what people say. Take a look now:

www.retireto.info/friendships/bookresources/

You will find interviews on a variety of retirement topics including friendship at retire-to.com. We will create links to the interviews relating to friendship on this web page as well.

---

13 Iris Tse report, myhealthnewsdaily.com, February 10, 2011

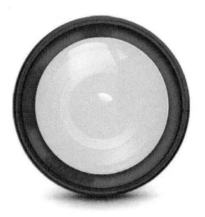

Part 2

So, now what?

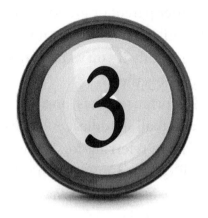

How Many Friends Am I Going to Need?

Wow. Did you read that list of research results? Sign me up. If friendship has that benefits package, I'm ready. Friendships are obviously important.

Friendships come in all sizes

Friendship, however, is not a one-size-fits-all proposition. As a result, the word "important" is elastic because it means different things for each level of friendship. Think about it a bit.

Let's say you have a buddy you play basketball with on a Saturday morning. You probably wouldn't share the details of your grandchild's troublesome behavior with him. On the other hand, you would be likely to talk about the same concerns with another parent or grandparent you know who has experienced similar issues. More importantly, you will discuss them more readily if you've been friends for a while, if you have a history together.

The issue of importance takes one tone when you are talking about basketball buddies and hits another note altogether when you're referring to fellow grandparents. If I change basketball courts, I might gather together a totally different team. On the other hand, I may want to keep taking the grandkids to a particular park because I can kick up that conversation again with the grandparent I met there. It would be hard to replace that individual with whom I'd already developed a rapport.

Basketball is not what makes the difference here. Rather, the difference is the level of connection. You are closer to the grandparent when it comes to discussing grandchild issues. You have a connection. Grandparenting is a more closely held, important issue to you than basketball.

Wasn't that spoken like a true grandparent? If I were more in tune with basketball, the situation might very well be reversed. Basketball might be more important to me, and I would continue to go back to the same venue because I was building a team, not just a collection of acquaintances for a pickup game. This role reversal doesn't belittle the point: People have a hierarchy of rapport that depends on the value they place on certain topics.

The hierarchy continues to at least four levels in my estimation. Marital or couple issues may take a higher position, along with other concerns that carry some vulnerability. It takes a level of mutual history before you share details about things like worries, disappointments, or life goals.

Topic hierarchy

If you map these discussion topics as a pyramid, at the bottom are the "safe" ones like the weather. You can usually count on everybody being discontented with the weather for some reason. Generally, you can't keep the weather a secret either. The weather is not personal. We discuss safe topics with our social **contacts**.

Add traffic to the safe topic list. Holiday preparation status, vacations, how cute the kids or grandkids are, grocery prices, coming movies, and where you can get discounts are all topics for social contacts—stuff you can talk about without looking around to see who is listening.

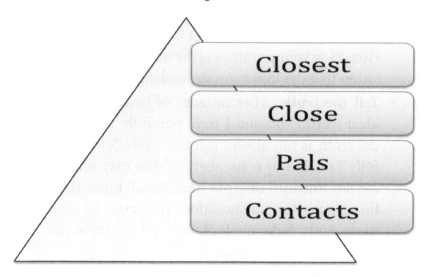

Pals, on the other hand, get into issues. Why do you think the hero did that? You don't just express curiosity about coming movies—you issue invitations. You have dinner with pals. You party with pals. You share exercise jaunts, go to events together and play cards or games. Pals laugh together.

The development of your close and closest friends is more complex, so let's look at those in more detail.

Close friends require a shared past, a one-on-one personal history. You can be a little more vulnerable with a close friend because you trust that person. Trust takes time to build.

If you've not done so in awhile, review with me the underpinnings of trust. You'll see why building it takes time. Put bluntly, there is quite a lot to it. But as I keep reminding my grandson: Nothing worth doing is easily done. You and I have learned these truths about trust. To garner trust you strive to

- **Do what you say.** Even if follow-through requires only a small thing, you and I know you can't blow off what you promised. A promise small to you may seem huge to another. Besides, big or little, not doing what you promised means you cannot be relied on in the future. Honoring your promises is the only way to gain a reputation that demonstrates dependability.

- **Tell the truth.** After decades of living in a less than ideal world, you and I have painfully discovered that the truth is not always just the truth. Speaking truthfully can lead to consequences that may make speaking an "untruth" easier to bear. We all know that truthful answers to some questions may even be cruel: "Do these pants make me look fat?" (OK. Maybe just men know that particular one.)

  Our motive may be pure. In some cases, for example, we may be trying to be kind! And steering straight toward kindness, we drive right into evasion. Sometimes, being discovered as evasive is like getting caught with pants half down. Not a pretty sight.

  And if the consequences of lying aren't bad enough, the consequences of a cover up can be worse. I've learned not to take that route.

- **Accept the truth.** Have you learned to be open to the truth? Sadly, the pants may indeed make me look fat. On the other hand, the witness testifying to fit may just be lashing out. Being open allows your friend to be truthful no matter how you might feel about it and lets you assess truth from anger.

  You don't have to hide your feelings, but you sometimes must put them in a secondary position. What you don't want to do is shrink from facts or hard topics or difficult decisions; doing so makes you less trustworthy.

- **Set boundaries.** On the other hand, you don't have to take continual abuse. You are allowed limits on what you are willing to discuss. You may find it helpful to tell your friend the limit. This disclosure is often a great relief because it takes the pressure off the other person to tell all. You are both allowed privacy.

- **Keep secrets.** If somebody tells you something in confidence, you and I know to keep that confidence. Discretion is the better part of valor. The only exception here is danger. If I'm putting myself or others in harm's way with the secrets I'm trying to keep, I want my friends to stand up for my best interest and against the harm. Seeking help is appropriate in such cases regardless of a request for secrecy.

- **Be consistent.** Friends need to know they can count on you being there when needed. That's not always easy, but the relationship benefits.

- **Be fair.** Demonstrating a strong moral ethic requires a variety of skills: trying to be neutral, being objective, and sticking to a single rather than double standard. It also means not asking some questions. For example, "Does this dress make me look fat?" We all know that the man's appropriate response is, "Does this shirt make me look stupid?"

What's wrong with the dress question? Well, it may be that the person asking the question wants different information. She actually might want to know whether she's still loved—how she looks in the dress doesn't matter. Because she's not asking the question she really wants answered, she's not being fair. Yes or no may not be the answer she wants to hear.

Do you think this list catches everything? I don't claim to be definitive here. I do know that what I've identified will take time. What do you consider important to building and keeping trust? What have been your experiences of broken or damaged trust?

Because of the trust level, shared activities are more extensive. You don't just go to a concert with a close friend; you may even go on vacation together. For example, we go to our friend Lanette's house overnight and joke about her providing the best B & B in the state. Lanette and my wife and I raised our daughters together. We are close. Actually more than close.

Closest friends start by being close and become even more involved, as we have with Lanette.

Discussion topics with your closest friends may include dreams, ambitions, desires, cares, and concerns, which are more intimate and personal. These issues touch on identity.

And, therein, lies the core of intimacy: touch. You not only "keep in touch," you "are in touch." You reach out to feel what the other feels, to hear and see and be in the world you share with each other. You can open up about your pain, remorse, guilt, joy, and pleasure. You are more vulnerable to your closest friends. You trust them to have your welfare at heart.

The intimacy you share with your closest friends does not necessarily involve sex. I am strongly in favor of being an intimate friend before having sex, however. That way sex becomes another way of showing and celebrating the level of closeness in the relationship, of being in touch. But sex is definitely not required to have a closest friend. On the other hand, if one of your closest friends is your spouse, wouldn't sex be a perfect way to celebrate the uniqueness of that relationship?

Marriage is not required of a closest friend either. However, I find that living with my wife helps nurture our strong relationship. That being said, cohabitation may not be needed between closest friends. Because I am married, because I do live in the same household with her, I'm definitely biased.

But I digress. Using the pyramid image, we have four groups: contacts, pals, close, and closest. They are separated with imprecise and fluid boundaries. What becomes clear, however, is that the level on the pyramid acts as a "volume control" for discourse.

You can talk to a lot of people about the weather. Those conversations are short. You're not making commitments. You don't have to worry about trust levels. You don't have to be very empathetic to commiserate about the heat.

You are not going to talk to a lot of people about your life dreams though. That would take too much time. It's not just the time it takes to have the one conversation, it's all the time required to build the level of trust needed to have those conversations in the first place.

You don't have conversations about some things that are out of your comfort zone. Desires, needs, concerns, angers, hurts, and grief are subjects limited to friends on the top of the pyramid. Such matters are hard to talk about because you are vulnerable and, therefore, you share them only with someone you can trust. Building that level of comfort takes time.

What it boils down to, then, is that you do different things with people in your social network depending on the level of intimacy you've developed.

The reverse is true as well. If you want to have someone to talk about your life dreams with, you spend more time to develop that relationship. Your investment varies with the level of need. You control the "volume."

The pyramid represents this volume. At the bottom we acknowledge far more people than at the top. We have a few friends we identify as our closest, probably more as close friends, hopefully many pals and, likely, a large number of social contacts.

And while I've tried to characterize these levels, I fully recognize the differences are not cast in stone. Firefighters, police officers, and military personnel put themselves in harm's way every day for people they have never met. Even though they obviously demonstrate caring, they may not be among your close or closest friends. At least they would not be there as friends; they would be there because, as firefighters or police officers, they are doing their jobs.

Doctors and other healthcare workers may show caring as well. So attending to someone's welfare is not exclusive to close or closest friends. But caring is crucial in intimate relationships.

Friendships are fluid

Another way to represent friendships is by showing connections as a line that allows the intensity to move back and forth depending upon factors such as proximity and shared experiences, as well as mutual respect and common values.

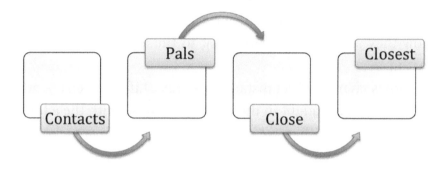

Friendships change. I had close friends in graduate school. We took separate career paths and spent decades conversing almost exclusively via Christmas newsletters. This past year we started getting reacquainted again. In other words our relationship for a time was at the right (closest) end of the scale, it moved over to the left (contacts) and now is moving to the right again.

The distance, in this case, does not seem to matter. We are becoming reacquainted with old friends from a variety of places around the country.

The gym my wife and I belonged to for years closed. Crys and I had made close friends in the water aerobics class there. Seeing one another four or five days a week encouraged conversation and caring. And because the class was demanding, the friendship had a "foxhole" feel;

we commiserated over levels of effort, tired muscles, new exercise demands, and on and on.

The foxhole disappeared when the gym closed. The locker room closeness vanished. Now we see our friends at funerals and for an occasional lunch. While we were at the gym, the relationships moved toward the right; now they are moving, regrettably, to the left. Proximity is a factor.

> *The goal is to keep your pyramid populated.*

Times change. Circumstances change. Life happens. And friendships get caught in the flux—they move with the effort put into them. When we spend more time with somebody, the relationship usually moves to the right on the scale. When we don't invest time, it can easily drift to the left.

Think about where your friends are located in the pyramid hierarchy or on the scale. I think the pyramid represents a series of goals and describes the levels of intimacy and discourse. The goal is to keep your pyramid populated.

In the flow of friendship, we should seek to have a few on the right, some in the middle categories, and more on the left. By keeping the pyramid well populated, occasional shifts in location by individuals won't affect the general result.

How do I even start making friends?

Faced with the reality of losing friends in retirement, some people have a hard time moving forward. Don't be discouraged. In the back of the closet you've stored some gear that can help you on the way. You may have forgotten it was there, but we can rummage around and find it again. Here are some reminders.

The first starts with the notion that your experiences with friends during your lifetime have formed your understanding friendship. The key word in the sentence, however, is *lifetime*. The concept of "lifetime" is pivotal to your success.

Friendship is not something you can be done with. "Well, I finished that!" Friendship is something you continually have to cross off and put back on your to-do list. You've been at it awhile; you need to keep at it if you want continuing results.

I don't care how many times the band I play in has successfully performed that song, if we do not invest ourselves through rehearsal, the next performance will not fare as well as previous ones. You have to put time in to get results, and you have to keep at it. Rehearsal is never over.

A performance may appear spontaneous, but it is not. Every minute of the act is carefully crafted. Like friendship, it takes time, planning, and practice. But friendship is not an act. It is far more vital. So, shouldn't the effort you put into it be even more? Here are two things to help you not be anxious:

- **Remember you have had a friend and been a friend before.** Friendship is part of your life's experience. So keep in mind that making more friends is entirely possible because you have done it before. You may have to brush up on a few details, but you have the T-shirt and, probably, the action figure to boot. You've been there before; you can do it again. Remember the Patronus, that magic guardian that materialized at Harry Potter's command. Harry Potter said to Hermione that he knew he could make the Patronus because he'd seen himself do it already!

- **Be persistent.** The final reminder is one about engagement. You did not start out knowing how to be a friend and have a friend. It took time and effort. You will not succeed this time unless you are willing to spend both. You have a challenge ahead. You have to invest yourself in meeting it.

You spent the years from age one until fourth or fifth grade learning how to move from parallel play to grasping the idea of teamwork. Reaching each milestone on the friendship trail took time. Why should the coming effort be different?

If you've been at the same job for some time where friends came as part of the territory, you may not have had to exercise the whole array of friend-making skills recently. After all, because it was a workplace, your potential friends were as close as the next seat in the lunchroom, a cubby over, or standing next to you, holding the frame up while you attached it to the building.

So, cut yourself some slack. You *can* rev up those skills again.

Like an investment, you benefit by making continued deposits over the long haul. The rewards are proportional to the effort. On one end of the spectrum, you have jotting down a status on your Facebook page and on the other, marriage. The more you put in, the more you get out.

Friendship takes time also because you have to nourish and hydrate what you plant. The more plants in the house, the more tending time it takes. This is a good thing!

One last point: Establishing new friendships begins with you taking initiative. You made friends at work partly because interaction with people turned out to be a sort of happy coincidence of being at a workplace. With retirement, the coincidence disappears. You're going to have to take steps to re-create the environment to make friends. Remember the fish bowl?

Your secret is to focus on these vital things:

- You can do it.
- It may take a while.
- You have to take charge.

So, where do you start? Think of this effort as having five parts. To grow your network of friends, you have to

- Find 'em
- Meet 'em
- Make 'em
- Keep 'em
- Love 'em

But before we can start down that road, we need to do a short refresher on the skills needed to develop and maintain any type of relationship.

For You

Did you find the pyramid and chart helpful? Take a look now:

www.retireto.info/friendships/bookresources/

Let's see how well they describe the communication levels you have with your friends. I've provided the simplest of forms you can use to talk about what you and your friends talk about.

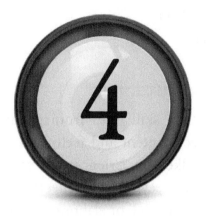

Sharpen Your Saw

Steven Covey, author of *The 7 Habits of Highly Effective People*, pointed out that having the right tools—and in good condition—makes a difference to the outcome. So before you tackle that building project, do as he said and "sharpen your saw."

Making friends requires some skills, which you can practice and get good at. Whether you are trying to meet people, make friends, or keep them, certain positive behaviors help. Of course, negative behaviors can upset the apple cart too.

In this chapter let's look at skills that will help you grow your network of fun and support throughout retirement. Musicians aren't the only ones who need to practice! Here are a few skills you will need:

- Listening well
- Making rejection work for you

- Paying attention
- Fighting fair

Practice active listening

Active listening is a skill born from genuine empathy. In essence you reflect content and feeling to demonstrate you understand the talker's experience. You are reflecting to the speaker: "I heard you say...." This reflection gives the speaker a chance to affirm, correct, or elaborate on the material he or she is attempting to convey.

An important element of active listening is your participation. You want the speaker to sense that you are engaged. Your body language is important. Keep eye contact and not only face the speaker, but also lean toward him or her. You want to understand the feeling message, as well as the thinking message.

You can further demonstrate you are engaged by restating a summary. Asking clarifying questions can also help identify central points or ideas and give the speaker the chance to examine other perspectives. Done well, active listening can bring hidden assumptions to light where, once in focus, they can be tested for validity.

Now that you've gotten the basic goals and ideas, let's try some active listening.

This is where you turn to me, keep eye contact, lean in and say,

Let me see if I've got it all. You think it is important to understand the experience of the talker, to listen carefully for what is said and felt. Is that right? Oh, and by the way, you want to try it out right now.

Bingo! You got it!

In addition to these tips, blogger Susie Cortright adds at least three very important rules:

- **Minimize external distractions:** TVs, phones, iPods can distract from the conversation. You may even need to move to a quieter place.
- **Minimize internal distractions:** This conversation is not about *you*. Don't let your point of view, ideas, conclusions, pet peeves, or even solutions get in the way. Try not to make assumptions about the speaker's thoughts.
- **Focus on what the speaker is saying:** Try not to think about what you are going to say next. The conversation will follow a logical flow after the speaker makes his or her point.[14]

Steven Covey conveyed the principle succinctly:

Seek first to understand, then to be understood.[15]

Reframe rejection

Here we are, way past junior high and still talking about rejection. Sadly enough, you will still be rejected. And now that you are putting yourself "out there" to meet people, you may find yourself rejected more. You may not get selected for a team, you might be left out of the group invited on a trip, you may feel your contribution was not valued.

But remember these key points, and you'll be able to get off the sidelines and back into the game:

---

14 "10 Tips to Effective & Active Listening Skills," by Susie Michelle Cortright, an undated blog post at the Power to Change website (powertochange.com). Published on or before December, 2012.
15 *The 7 Habits of Highly Effective People*, by Steven R. Covey. First copyright © 1989 by Steven R. Covey; published by Simon and Schuster.

- **Everybody gets rejected.** This truth is the hardest to learn because you often see only your rejection. Just because you were the last chosen for the team does not mean others did not feel rejected along the way for not being chosen first or not being selected for the "good" team. You can't duck; life brings rejection. In fact, by saying some of the things I have in this list, I may be rejecting your pet notion about rejection. Take that!

- **Rejection feels personal.** Knowing that everybody else feels rejected does not make the feeling less painful to me or to you; it just means the problem is more widespread than we assume while we are focused on our own suffering. I do find it somewhat less painful, however, to know my heroes are not immune.

- **Rejection can be a catalyst for improving.** Abraham Lincoln did *not* get elected for government positions more often than he did get elected. Twelve publishers rejected J.K. Rowling's manuscript before the first *Harry Potter* book was accepted and published.

Michael Jordan has a famous quote about failure:

> *I've missed more than 9,000 shots in my career. I've lost almost 300 games. Twenty-six times, I've been trusted to take the game-winning shot and missed. I've failed over and over and over again in my life. And that is why I succeed.*[16]

That kind of attitude can transport you around or over the rejection and enable you to take the next steps.

When you don't get picked, often somebody else's expectations are driving the choice. If you realize that, the rejection could lead to a positive chain of events. Making the experience positive depends on the steps you take. Try these:

---

16 Michaeljordanquotes.org

- **Seek answers.** Business consultants encourage compa-
  nies seeking to improve their products to ask the people
  who did not buy why they didn't. More information is
  better, even if the information is unwelcome. Can you
  come up with the right solution if you don't know the
  problem?

  Unfortunately, answers may not be forthcoming for
  you. There may be a disconnect between the person
  who passed on the rejection and the one who actually
  made the decision. Sometimes you can't connect with
  the person who actually decided. Your contact may not
  have the knowledge to give you an answer.

  Ideally, the answers would not be anything you can do
  something about. The company may have had too many
  to choose from—500 applicants! Or they were seeking
  to expand their skill base and already had enough of
  yours: *We have quilts. We need tapestries!*

- **Evaluate.** Rejection does hurt, and rejection by some
  people can hurt more than by others. Those feelings are
  normal, but don't let them delay your efforts. A helpful
  way to move on is to ask whether the evaluations of
  others are true. Do you need to improve in order to be
  chosen? If so, how do you improve? You could try again
  later after more training or a change in approach.

  The evaluation might also lead you to the conclusion
  that you don't need improvement—you need a new audience. J.K. Rowling's original *Harry Potter* manuscript
  was rejected multiple times because publishers did not
  think children's books, especially long ones, would sell.
  She continued to submit the work to others. One casu-
  ally gave the manuscript to his eight-year-old daughter.
  She read it and wanted more. The publisher made the
  deal. Rowling succeeded because her book finally got

to the person who could evaluate it fairly—a child, not
a publisher.

- **Try again.** Please don't attempt to avoid rejection. Don't
let the fear of failure get the better of you. Try again. Re-
cast your effort; take steps to improve. Having another
chance is a gift. Give it to yourself; you're the only one
who can. Then, grab it.

Pay attention to significance

My wife says I'm terribly hard to shop for. On the other hand, I
can usually find something for her that not only surprises, but
also it delights. I attribute the difference to paying attention.

Whoops. Did I just say my wife doesn't pay attention? Well,
yes and no. In this situation, she's not as good at it. Her brain
focuses on very different things than mine. In particular she
waits until Christmas or birthday time to pay attention to
what would be a good gift. Often this means she's way too
late.

I try to watch all the time, which means I can often find some
idea to explore in plenty of time to do something about it. In
March I discover some gardening thing she values because
she's doing gardening then. Had I waited until Christmas, the
right gift would have remained a mystery.

But finding out in March, I have another problem—
remembering. It is very easy for me to forget the March
discovery when I'm shopping in December. Purchasing the
item in March doesn't help much because I can easily forget
where I hid it. (I still haven't found the book I purchased for
Randy last September, and we're due to celebrate Christmas
with his family in two days!)

Another reason my wife has a hard time shopping for me
is that shopping in general is not high on her priority list. It's

not on mine either, but I also value gift giving as a means of showing love. Crys values presence more than presents as her expression of love.

But the idea here is not so much how you show love or ways you expect to receive love. We'll focus on that a little more in *Chapter 9: Love 'em*. The focus here is on paying attention to significance. Can you name the five things your golfing buddy enjoys besides golf? Here are key things to watch for:

- What makes his eyes light up?
- Does she move any faster going for this rather than that?
- What issues motivate her to take a stand?
- Does he complain about staying awake nights because of this?

Knowing what is significant to your friends is like figuring out just where they are ticklish. You have to poke them here and there and watch the result.

Here are some guidelines for tending to your relationship:

- **Anticipate**: It is Christmas time. What does your friend do to prepare? A more telling example might be family visits. Your friend's brother is coming to town. Is this a good thing or a bad thing? Why? You can learn what is significant to your friend by paying attention to coming events.
- **Avoid distraction**: Listen and learn, Grasshopper. You can't be off woolgathering and hope for success. Besides, your friend needs to know you care. Look attentive and interested!
- **Ask questions**: You may not always get an answer; but when gaps in what you know also inhibit your ability to help, you can always ask.

- **Listen—don't just talk**: Rule #1: It is not about you. The goal is to learn what is significant to your friend, not you.
- **Don't assume**: Just because you "always do it that way" does not mean your friend has, or even wants to.
- **Try not to be alarmed**: You may not think lighting a paper bag filled with dog poop is a great practical joke. I don't either! But finding out your friend once thought this was hilarious is the kind of surprise we both need to be prepared for. No wincing. This is your friend we're talking about. (You might want to circle back later to see if the joke is still being repeated.)

Ultimately, these practices boil down to paying attention and tending to your friend. You are not watching passersby, you are not checking your phone, and you most definitely are not trying to figure out what to say next. You are attentive.

You need to "check in" when you are spending time with your friend. Turn on the "I'm with my friend now" switch, and turn off whatever you were doing earlier. This is together time. When you feel yourself wandering, say to yourself "Stop. Watch. Listen." Move your attention back to being with your friend. You have to be fully present to your friend to understand what is significant to him or her.

Fight fair

Do you run from conflict? Others try to battle to the death. Still others retreat into their shell. These responses are autonomic. They are as close to us as breathing. When faced with danger, our response is flight, fight, or freeze.

The problem, of course, is that the conflict does not go away. Although over time the urgency may dissipate, being less upset about an issue does not mean that it has gone away.

And, worse, it may roar back at a later, completely unexpected time. Fighting fair is an essential skill for maintaining relationships.

The first rule about fighting fair: You generally can't fix anything by yelling at each other. If you need some time to settle your feelings, do two things: Agree to return to the issue at a later time and then take a break.

You may not be able to achieve the two things if you are so angry you have to throw things. So, try to have the conversation about steps prior to a conflict. Your friend may be just as happy to duck until the throwing stops. But you need to come back to words to resolve the issue.

Exaggeration does not help. Nobody could feel that bad over what happened. Oops. You may not want to generalize either. Avoid these words:

Everybody
Nobody
Always
Never
Can't
Won't
…and variations.

Try to be factual. "I saw the ball fall on his head" is far different from "You threw the ball at his head." And don't even bother to add, "You are cruel." Adding blame or attributing unwarranted motivations just aggravates the situation.

None of this happened last year. As far as this disagreement goes, it happened in a void, today. Bringing up old wounds just opens them and adds layers of resentment and hurt, which does not help. Once you have resolved a conflict, let it go. No need to visit it again—ever.

Fighting fair, paying attention, making rejection work for you, and listening well are all valuable skills. They are important when making pals and essential to maintaining close and intimate relationships.

You have an advantage with new friends: surprise. They don't know about the mistakes you may have made in the past. So, put your best foot forward; keep these skills in mind as you seek new friends.

For You

Skills are useful when actively practiced. It is also helpful to remind yourself of the subtleties. Take a look now:

www.retireto.info/friendships/bookresources/

I've included a wonderful two-page cheat sheet on the art of active listening prepared by the National Aging Information & Referral Support Center.

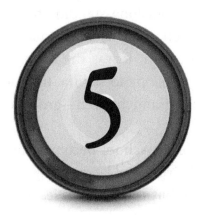

Find 'em

Where do I find new friends?

This part of the task starts out looking incredibly easy. You find friends by going to places where friends hang out.

Duh!

So, the first step is to list places where *you* might meet friends.

Wow. That sounds simple. What am I missing? you say.

I don't want to belittle the effort here. A lot of people have reached retirement without ever having to go out and look for a friend. They've been in environments that provided everything needed for friend-finding. Let me explain.

At first, parents did the front-end grunt work by making sure you got to know the kids of *their* friends. In our household, spending time with our long-standing friend Lanette meant our daughter, Ellen, had a ready-made companion in Lanette's daughter, Erin. It was the beginning of a lifelong friendship, and I'm happy to say the tradition continues, as their children—our grandchildren—are becoming friends, as well.

As kids grow older, school becomes the source for new friends. Boys and girls—and later, young men and women—may come and go, but the possibilities are there for lasting friendships. Classrooms, the lunchroom, and the playground are the growing-up versions of the water cooler.

Finally, there is the workplace—often more than one—which, as we've said, provides ample opportunities to meet and greet and make friends.

Retirement may change this equation dramatically. You may not be able to rely on your mom to introduce you to the children of her friends. You probably don't even want to do that at this time of your life!

The bottom line is that you have to be a little more involved in finding a "water cooler" that suits! So, while the steps seem simple, don't shortchange them. Finding venues you value might be difficult.

Cast your net wide. You don't have to use all the ideas presented here, but you need a variety of options that make you feel comfortable.

At the beginning, don't be too critical of your list of places. You may try out a venue that is not immediately to your liking, but friends you make there could make it more appealing when all is said and done. Don't rule out anything, at first.

Step 1: Decide where to go

Take a nice big sheet of paper and start making lists or circles.
I like circles:

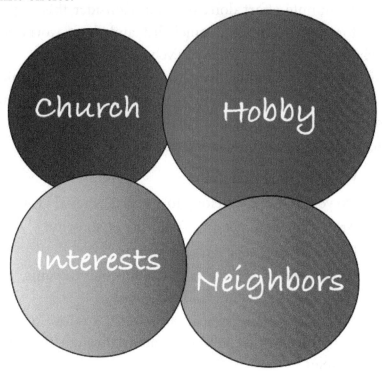

Let's start with the easy ones. Where have you made friends
before?

- Church or temple
- Neighborhood
- School
- Club
- Activity

Some places probably come quickly to mind. Then, expand
the list. Have you had more than one hobby or lived in more
than one location? List those also in any category where you
have multiples. Two schools? Three neighborhoods?

This inventory may take you all of five minutes the first time. Don't worry about that. You may need to invest more time on this step later, particularly if the results of the easy five-minute effort don't pan out. Consider this step as brainstorming. Compile a quick list and don't worry too much about evaluating what you've written.

If you are having difficulty getting started or are returning to this list to do more work, think of the places where you are vested already. You may not currently have friends in these places, but they may be starting points:

- Where do you exercise?
- Do you or did you belong to any professional groups?
- Are you or were you in a fraternity or sorority?
- Do you belong to a veterans group?
- What about a service organization like Kiwanis, Jaycees, Rotary, Civitan, or Lions Club?
- Are there small groups, short-term studies, or special projects you can participate in through church or temple?

Get them on the list.

Don't forget work!

But, Ed! Didn't we just come from there? Isn't that where we lost all our friends?

Yes, you did. Maybe not *all* of our friends from work. But even if they've not called you, you probably have some folks there with whom you would still want to keep in touch. For Pete's sake—I am good friends with the young man I trained to take my last job! His success shoved me out the door (kicking and yelling "yippee" all the way).

Just because your friends disappeared last week doesn't mean they have to stay MIA. Is there someone you want to reach out to next week? You don't have to limit yourself to the last job, either. Who are possibilities from previous jobs?

Don't forget the schools you attended, your hometown, or other locations where you've lived. Most of us come from someplace else. You may want to evaluate whether or not you want to reach out (or should we say "back") to those places.

Don't be discouraged if you have only a few circles. You can—and may want to—add more. Where would you like to go next? Maybe some of the circles on your list are organizations you would like to be a part of. Or some of the circles may represent activities you've always wanted to try. Curiosity leads to new possibilities.

If you are not exercising now, maybe a membership to a fitness center or the Y may be in order.[17] You can kill two birds with one stone: You might end up being more fit *and* making friends. My wife and I go out to lunch periodically with people from our former water aerobics class; the center where we worked out together closed, but we still stay in touch. We shared the struggle of keeping healthy, and we still laugh together!

If you don't belong to an organization, maybe it's time to join. Sign up with a professional organization, for example. In my case, I don't develop software 40 hours per week any more, but that does not mean I've suddenly lost interest in the latest gizmos, tricks, jargon, and ideas. And the people. These are my kind of folks; why abandon them?

I taught courses for professional data processing personnel in systems analysis and project management for a decade. Paul Saunders, retired now, was the man I worked for and the

---

17 Did you know that some retirement medical plans include memberships in *Silver Sneakers* at the Y? Our Medicare Advantage provider gives us free memberships to this nationwide fitness program for older adults.

co-teacher for these courses. He still hosts a monthly AITP (Association of Information Technology Professionals), meeting at his house. Paul keeps his hand in. You don't have to be doing the business every day all day to be interested.

You know, you may have acquired some wisdom and experience along the way. Sharing that may be very helpful. Paul's decades of management, systems work, and training is a resource that can be a positive influence on the people in AITP. He can still make a contribution. What contribution can you make?

I knew a gentleman a long time ago who claimed he was getting to that stage in life to be a "Sage." I don't remember the other stages he had mapped out. I just remember he thought he'd reached the place where he could be the mentor, the coach, and the advocate. What could you coach? Who might you mentor? Who among people you know needs guidance and support? In what topic would you have the expertise to be a mentor?

I would be remiss if I did not include family in this list. Please, don't take your family for granted. I know friends are easier because they don't come with all the history the folks in your family do. Friends don't start out knowing your secrets.

On the other hand, the history that comes with family can be positive. I remember great Thanksgiving, Easter, and Christmas get-togethers. Laughter. Smiling. Teasing. Watching football. Playing cards. These are all positive activities to build on. Consider spreading this wealth to the next generation, including your nieces and nephews and their children. So, add a family circle. See where it leads.

My absolute, all-time best friend is my wife. I don't have to have a "spouse" circle to remind me to keep in contact. Do you?

The first step then is to make a list of places where you have, or could, or would like to find friends.

Step 2: Identify people

You don't become friends with a hobby. You become friends with people doing that hobby. So, where you can, go back to your list and add names if you know them. For example, if you're interested in golf, write in that golf-playing neighbor's name. If you're starting a garden, add the names of the couple down the street with the big flowerbed.

Think about the challenge here. If the objective is to be friendly and perhaps befriend someone else, the sooner you can identify who might be a candidate, the closer you will be to your objective.

Start with your activities, organizations, or groups you noted in the circles. Head a blank sheet of paper for each of those. Under each heading write the names of people you know or would like to know better. Don't worry if the listing is not long now. The numbers may grow as you move forward.

For You

Sometimes a log is the easiest solution. Take a look now:

www.retireto.info/friendships/bookresources/

For this chapter I've included a simple one-page form you can duplicate as needed to build a file of interests, activities and ideas. And I've included a few questions to get you started.

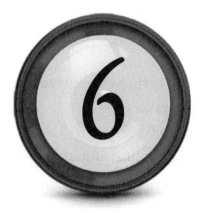

Meet 'em

*H*ow do I go about meeting new people?

It is not enough to know where to go. You gotta get there! You've done the trip planning. Now start driving. If the previous activity was about the "where," this one is about the "how."

So, just how do we start driving? What do we do? Go to church, button-hole somebody, and say, "*Hi, I'm Ed. Wanna be my friend?*"

We wouldn't do that. Right? Here's what we can do:

Step 1: Identify activities

Make another list of things you enjoy or would like to do.

- Golfing?
- Playing cards?

- Being with animals?
- Gardening?
- Cooking?
- Taking photos, perhaps through a telescope?
- Listening to speakers?
- Seeing art exhibits?
- Singing, playing an instrument, or attending concerts?

These activities provide the means for meeting folks. Here's our favorite:

Early in our married life, my wife and I moved 2,000 miles away from home to attend graduate school. We knew no one. We definitely felt isolated! The advice we were given? Kids and dogs. Dogs and kids. You have to walk the dog or the baby or take the preschooler to the playground. People will greet you! You're one of the safe ones, because you have a cute dog—or a cute kid. Kids and dogs—a good way to meet your neighbors.

What might your to-do list look like? You can start with the dreams you had for retirement. When I planned my retirement, I promised myself I would learn more about photography and take better pictures. So I added photography classes to my list. One instructor turned out to be a neighbor, and now we're working on other projects together. Bingo. A "two-for"!

Sometimes these activities come with their own venue. If so, you can go back and add a circle or worksheet for that group. Sometimes activities don't come with a particular setting. If they do not, you can connect those dots in Step 2.

When you are listing activities, pay attention to your internal "comfort meter." Some folks are just not at ease stepping forward and introducing themselves or walking up to a group and asking to join in an already engaged activity. In some situations, doing so might also be rude; we certainly don't want to start off a potential relationship by alienating everyone.

If you are more reticent, then you may want to join in activities that expect newcomers. Our water aerobics class was fun, and it was always open to newcomers. That group included enough outgoing folks so that any stranger was likely to feel welcome without having to step forward to meet folks.

Joining a Sunday school class or attending a Wednesday night church dinner would put you in a place where people would recognize a "newbie" in the group. The folks there will likely welcome you and find ways to get you involved gradually.

One final word about expectations: Don't pick a large group. For example, if you walked into a worship setting with 600 people, you may not meet anybody. Those 600 people may have no way of recognizing the newcomer! However, if you joined a small group at the same church or synagogue, the story should be different.

Step 2: Join up!

Think intelligently about the people side of the equation. You can find a lot of activities that do not require other people. But if you're intentional about making friends, you want activities that involve others.

Exercise. Take a class at a local gym, senior center, or community fitness facility. Organize a lunchtime walking group at work (whether you still work there or not).

Volunteer. Offer your time or talents at a hospital, place of worship, museum, community center, charitable group, or other organization. You can form strong connections when you work with people who have mutual interests.

Join a faith community. Take advantage of special activities and get-to-know-you events for new members.

Attend community events. Get together with a group of people working toward a goal you believe in, such as an election or the cleanup of a natural area. Find a group with similar interests in an activity, such as auto racing, gardening, reading, or making crafts.

Go to school. Take a college or community education course to meet people who have similar interests. Wouldn't hurt to meet younger people, either.

Try "meetups." Young folks do it by sending mass text messages: "Come to the train station at 7:00." You can do it by looking at the bulletin boards posted at churches, schools, recreation centers, park centers, and so on.

People also get together through meetup.com. The website works nationwide and might help you find or establish meetings. These meetups can be about anything and everything:

Crafts	Hobbies	Movies	Ethics
Classes	Entertainment	Schools	Foreign Film
Games	Science Fiction	Swing Dance	Backpacking
Issues	Lifestyle	Songwriting	Books
Language	Literature	Motorcycles	Hair Styling
Outdoors	Hiking	Biking	Karaoke
Pets	Photography	Writing	Beatles
Sports	Tech	Knitting	Put yours here!

Get the idea? Didn't find a group that looks good? The website will let you start one of your own.

Step 3: Put places, interests, people together

So, we now have three lists: places of interest, people, and activities. Where do these three lists cross over? Where do your interests intersect with groups you've joined (or want to) and other venues? I may not be able to play golf at the church or temple, but can I volunteer to cook? Cooking doesn't happen every day, but the opportunities are frequent. Do some exploration.

In one church, the "Double-Nickel Club," folks 55 or older, meets regularly and some folks in the group play cards. Because the group meets on Tuesday during the day, I never paid attention. I was always working. Guess what, I can now meet on Tuesday—I'm retired!

Ed, was that your church? Well… No. You don't always have to be a member to join in an activity.

Some churches do things you like to do and others don't. I've played with a bluegrass band for over 30 years that carries the name of a church I don't belong to any longer. The band is one of the reasons I have so much experience with nursing homes.

Think about each of the locations you've scouted and ask yourself the following questions:

- What can I do there?
- How often can I do it?
- Will the activity help me get to know folks?

Start with the intersections that make the most sense and move on to Step 4.

Step 4: Set goals

Why do we need goals?

An old adage convinces me I need to think through something far enough ahead to set goals. The maxim goes like this:

Shoot at nothing; hit nothing!

If you don't have goals, it is much harder to reach a successful solution. Setting goals will help you gain clarity about what *exactly* you want to achieve. Hopping around, trying this and that, may get results but may also waste a lot of time.

It's better to spend the time getting to the desired result than going through a series of false starts. If you give a million monkeys a chance, one may write a Shakespearean play. But 999,999 of them won't. You need to take aim.

Goals can be motivators. Having a goal is sometimes the "alarm clock" that starts your day. The goal gives you places to go and things to do!

Goals also help you focus on the result and eliminate distractions. Yes, you may want to sleep instead. But if you do, you will know what you missed—because you had a goal. This in turn will help you be accountable to yourself.

I believe you are getting the picture. I'm a fan of goals. But I'm also a fan of being your own boss. You don't have to be a Type A personality to set goals and follow through. You do have to replace another one of those things you left behind at work: the boss. Go for it! Being your own boss is an American dream. Now is your chance.

I also advocate SMART goals. SMART goals are far and away the easiest form of goal setting and exactly suited for what you need to do next.

SMART goals have five very specific parts; a SMART goal is

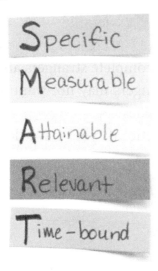

I will illustrate a SMART goal by giving several examples related to our task at hand. Later, I'll talk more about SMART goal practices and suitability.

Your SMART goals can start at one of two points. You can start with locale or action. Here is a SMART goal connected to a venue:

By next Wednesday, I will take a plate of cookies to the Harris family down the street. I bet the kids love peanut butter cookies.

This is a SMART goal because it is

- **Specific**: A plate of cookies and Harris family are very specific.
- **Measurable**: I'm planning on one plate and one family.
- **Attainable**: I'm planning on taking only one plate to only one family.
- **Relevant**: Folks like cookies and if they're good cookies, you're golden!

- **Time-bound**: I'm planning to do this by next Wednesday.

What happens if I don't know the Harris family?

Well, partly, it depends on how brave you are. Some people would have no problem going up to complete strangers and offering them cookies. But some strangers may not want to accept cookies. Hmm. Maybe not cookies?

You might need a different tactic if you have less information. Let's try again.

Next Saturday, I will take a plate of cookies to the neighborhood picnic. I'll ask my neighbor to introduce me to the people in the brick house. I think their name is Harris.

You have to start somewhere. A neighbor you know might become your champion, so to speak. If you are entirely new to the neighborhood, talk to your realtor or landlord. Find out about neighborhood watch groups, local clubs or organizations, picnic areas, neighborhood associations and parks.

Another place to start is with the activities. Again, here is a SMART goal:

By next week, I'll check with the community center I saw down the street to see if a garden club meets there.

You want to do gardening? A community center might sponsor a garden club. Your neighbor might know other folks who garden. (Your friends from work might also know folks who garden, but unless they live in your neighborhood, their information may not be helpful.)

Now let's move to the second part of Step 3: **Set multiple SMART goals.**

Come on. You won't make any progress if you limit yourself to one at a time. Be a little aggressive. You want your goals to provide a challenge. Try three to five to start. When you realize how easy making them really is, make more. What have you got to lose? Another hour of TV?

Let's get started. I challenge you to fill in the blanks on the following three SMART goals. Remember **S**pecific, **M**easureable, **A**ttainable, **R**elevant, **T**ime-bound:

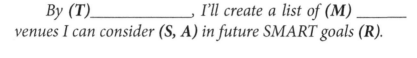

By (T)_____, I'll create a list of (M) _____ venues I can consider (S, A) in future SMART goals (R).

By (T)_____, I'll create a list of (M) _____ activities I can consider (S, A) in future SMART goals (R).

These are preliminary goals we set so we can set some goals so we can meet some folks. Simple.

You need to get past these two and move on. So, for your final step, set one more goal, please:

By (T)_____, I'll write (M) _____ SMART goals that will help me move forward with my challenge (S, A) of meeting new friends (R).

If you need some ideas to get started, take a look at the Appendix. You will find nearly two-dozen examples, plus more specific details about what constitutes a SMART goal.

Here are some tips for making your goal-setting more beneficial to you:

Consider the benefits

"I want to have a billion dollars" is a great goal but hardly specific enough to get you started. Though it might describe why you are making the effort. SMART goals supply the how.

Without the how, achieving results is harder.

It can't hurt to add a benefits statement, the "why," to your SMART goals. Doing so brings relevance into sharper focus.

*I will meet the Harris family next Wednesday **in order to** help me have a stronger social network.*

Write reminders

You might even write reminders of these benefits. Put the reminders on your to-do list or calendar. Make notes on the fridge. Reminders can encourage you to think and talk about the goals—again. It's all about taking one step at a time, again and again.

The world can interfere

When I was working, it always irked me that the boss wanted to know when I could have something finished. From her point of view, my timeline made a difference because the tasks she had in mind to follow the one I was doing couldn't even start until I was done. In the meanwhile she needed to tell the crew working on the next steps what to expect. How could she coordinate things without knowing?

You probably don't have the same kind of coordination problem. On the other hand, if you intend to take your best cookies to the neighborhood picnic next Saturday, you can't make them Sunday, the day after.

I realize SMART goals are not for everyone. They are a *means* to an end. In this case the end is *get out the door and meet folks*. If you have a better way to do that, go for it! I'm right behind you.

But if you find yourself on the couch or in front of the TV or playing too many computer games, use SMART goals. They can help you get out and about, meeting people.

If you've identified where you can make friends, have homed in on some activities you'd like to pursue and, if you've written some carefully crafted SMART goals to get you started, you've only one thing left to do.

Get started. Follow those SMART goals and...

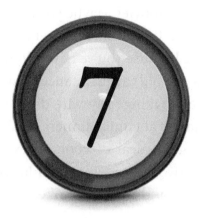

Make 'em

All you have to do now is make friends.

Will you have accomplished that after you complete your first five SMART goals?

Maybe.

But actually to move the relationship from a *"Hi"* to *"That was fun! Want to do it again?"* you may need some additional ideas. Despite the world's best book on pick-up lines, guys still walk away without a date because no magic words will make that date happen.

So, what are we to do?

Idea 1: Practice being invitational

Need a lunch break out? Are you going shopping? Want to go to the garden store? Do you wish you could ride your bike?

Want to see that new movie? Maybe you'd like to volunteer to work at that event at the community center but would really like an accomplice because you've never done it before. What if you took a new (or old) acquaintance along next time?

Want some help baking? My wife decided we needed to serve more vegetables at family dinners, so she asked another lady who had a great deal of cooking experience to help with recipes. The two got together, had lunch on the veggie dishes they created, and my wife walked away with help for the family dinner. She also walked away knowing she had deepened a relationship.

All these things are natural ways to have an excuse to be invitational. Here are a few phrases you can practice building into your lifestyle:

Let's get together and…
Come over and…
I was thinking about you and…
Let's go and…

Being invitational can help you think of yourself as someone who spends time with people. You don't have to be alone and won't be if you practice inviting people along.

Idea 2: Accept invitations

You are not the only one building a network. Invitations are a two-way street. When you're invited to a social gathering, say yes. Being open to invitation is just as important as being invitational.

Or, tit for tat, you can contact someone who recently invited you to an activity and return the favor.

Idea 3: Learn a new way to talk about yourself

Having a job gives you a great opening gambit in making new acquaintances.

Hi. I'm Ed. I have my own software company.

With that phrase, the dance begins. The classic rejoinders pop up: "Oh, really. Do you know Harriet? She is a software engineer." Conversation is started. The ice is broken. You can begin to move this fledgling friendship forward.

When you retire, just what do you say?

Hi. I'm Ed. I don't have a job.

What kind of response does that provoke? Probably not what I wanted! I cheated. When I retired, I started a new company:

Hi. I'm Ed. I am the cofounder of Retirement-U.

Hmm. Somehow, that does not seem to cut it either. Not many people start a new company (or want to) when they retire.

What you need is a new "elevator spiel." You know what an elevator spiel is, right? If you only had the time it takes to get from the fifth floor to the first, what would you say to sell your product? You might think of an elevator spiel as a bio or verbal business card, but I think it is more than that.

My friend Steve says to tell folks you are self-employed. You may not make any money, but at least people understand being self-employed. Steve has a point. If you meet someone randomly and not as part of your SMART goal system, you should have a way of talking about yourself that does not refer to work.

Steve found out that people don't understand what retirement is all about. You can't say

Hi. I'm Ed. I'm retired.

That doesn't work either because the word *retirement* actually has very negative definitions:

Withdrawal from one's occupation, business, or office
Leaving of job or career
Taken out of active circulation
Fall back, **retreat**, **depart**…

I get the feeling that some people become green with envy because *they* want to take naps, spend all their time on cruises, and play with their grandchildren all the time. Just like we do. Oh… and they think we have no money worries either.

Others seem to expect us to keel over at any moment.

Here, have a seat. Can I get that for you?

The envious lot view retired people as being disengaged. Retirees are no longer in the "real" world. After all they live in the fantasy land the envious ones dream about when they think of being retired. (Sigh)

At the very least they don't expect retirees to carry on a civilized conversation because we retirees are no longer involved or active in the work-a-day world as they are.

Negative connotations of retirement are still predominant in advertisements, comedy routines, and social discourse. As for me—I am not elderly, and I'm not closed for business, thank you very much!

So, what *do* you say?

Assuming the person you are addressing is one you want to cultivate as a friend, the advice I give boils down to a single thought: What do you want to accomplish with the conversation? You are headed somewhere; it is up to you to figure out where. So, for example, if you want to spark interest in having lunch some time, work backwards from there.

Problem: *We haven't had lunch in too long.*

Solution: *I think we owe it to ourselves to catch up.*

Qualifications: *Luckily, I'm retired, so I have a lot of flexibility in my schedule.*

Goal: *How 'bout I call you this afternoon to set a time?*

Elevator spiels have to vary. When you worked for a living, you might have had one elevator spiel for a potential investor and a different spiel for a prospective employer.

The retired person is no different. You don't have lunch with everybody. You could also suggest a golf game, card game, service project, or movie night.

In other words, an elevator spiel doesn't describe who you are as much as it helps move the relationship to a different level.

We've been out of touch; can we do lunch soon?

We had a great time at the last movie; I'm free Saturday night, so how about another movie?

I've killed off another rose bush. Can I call to set a time you could take a look at my surviving bushes?

One elevator pitch need not copy another. According to author Dan Pink, they don't have to sound or look alike, either. He claims six different ones:

1. The Question Pitch
2. The Rhyming Pitch

3. The Subject Line Pitch
4. The One-Word Pitch
5. The Twitter Pitch
6. The Pixar Pitch[18]

Obviously, the genre has changed due to the prevalence of electronic options. We are no longer limited to elevators.

This change is a good thing. It gives us all more options. I bet you have invited others to lunch via email. Well, what did the subject line say?

Idea 4: It is not always about you

Just so we're clear here: Even though we're talking about how important friendships are to us, being a friend is not about us. Being a friend is about the other person.

What can you do for the other person? What does he or she need? A ride to the airport? A sitter for the dog? A trip to the grocery?

Ralph Waldo Emerson may have said it best:

"If we would build on a sure foundation in friendship we must love friends for their sake rather than our own."

—Charlotte Brontë

The only reward of virtue is virtue; the only way to have a friend is to be a friend.

Idea 5: Cut everybody some slack

As hard as it may seem to imagine, sometimes people do not accept your invitations. Sometimes circumstances play a role. If you had to walk the whole three miles both ways

---

18 *To Sell Is Human,* by Dan Pink. Copyright © 2012 by Daniel Pink.

with snow up to your waistband and drifts as high as your head and it was cold enough to freeze your mustache, getting someplace might take a little longer! Just like Grampa going to school. You can't always do it.

Besides, you don't always know what is going on. If you need some slack sometimes, the other guy might too. You don't have the full picture. When you invite someone to lunch and he or she seems brusque in response, it could be that he was rushing out the door for an appointment or that she was not feeling well or….

I have a tendency to blame myself for whatever happens. A friend of ours from the pool had not been there regularly. I looked for what we—and in particular, what I—may have done that chased her off. Turns out her absence wasn't about us or about me. She had been overwhelmed because she had to put her husband in hospice care.

> "Be kind, for everyone you meet is fighting a hard battle."
>
> —Plato

Wow. Didn't I feel foolish? Can you spell "insensitive lout"? I hadn't known her husband was anywhere near that ill. Just how caring a friend was I?

The takeaway from this experience is that you need to circle back. Don't write off a person for a single negative response. Ask again later.

Idea 6: Grow your family

Back when I was in graduate school and we lived 2,000 miles from home, most of our acquaintances shared a problem: What would we do on holidays? Many of us had familiar traditions that included family, but those traditions could not be repeated so far from home.

As a group, we decided to celebrate special occasions with one another. So, we gathered together and made our favorite Thanksgiving (Christmas, Easter) dishes and shared a potluck meal. Our friends became a new "family." The whole experience was great. We substituted laughter and friendship and a feast for what might have been a solitary meal and, if not a lonely occasion, certainly a less festive one.

About ten years ago, when my daughter got married, we started the tradition again. We had family in the area we didn't see as often as we wanted, so we started what we call "Monday night dinner."

We rotated hosting and cooking chores among our daughter, Ellen, and her family; a life-long friend who lived two blocks away; and Crys' stepbrother, wife, and mother. We traded cooking something every Monday for cooking everything once in four Mondays. One week we would host; the next week would find us at our daughter's house, and on we would go around the circle, rotating kitchens. Fantastic. Yummy too.

Then things changed. Stepbrother and family moved. Our friend two blocks away moved. Hmm... do we continue Monday dinners? Where do we find more family?

My wife is used to that question. She used to say to her mother that she wanted a sister. Her mother told Crys that she was the lucky one because, as an only child, she could pick her own sister. So Crys did. She and Emma have been active friends since first grade.

So we started inviting our friends to Monday night dinner. After all, in graduate school the events and holidays were not limited to actual family. We extended our family then, we could do so now.

> *"Friends are family you get to choose."*
>
> —*Unknown*

Currently we have five regulars for dinner who are not family. Dave and Tom, a father-son duo, have been with us for eight years or so. Casey is a college student who was invited initially because she was new to town and friends with Crys' long-time friend, Emma. Clare, the fourth, is a dear friend from church who also plays fiddle with me at the nursing homes from time to time. And Amanda, a newer friend from church.

Each of these guests has tenure; they can keep the position for as long as they choose. But work schedules change, people move, interests migrate and students graduate. We have watched people come and go, and we expect things will change again in the future.

What will remain the same, however, is that we will continue making friends and deepening relationships with our chosen "family" on Monday nights.

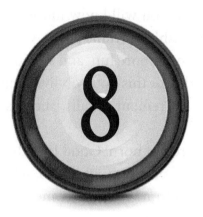

Keep 'em

You've made friends, but you're not finished. You need to set up a way to keep this quest for new friends going in your life. You are not solving a one-time problem. You are focusing on a series of activities that work because you continually give them energy. Making friends is an ongoing series of cookies and greetings, of neighborhood picnics, of classes at church or temple. Such activities are worth the effort all the time.

Setting a SMART goal is not the same thing as accomplishing the mission. The long-range task is to create a "friend-making" mindset. You have friends because you are friendly, not just last week, and not just tomorrow when you deliver the cookies. You are friendly all the time. You are a friendly person.

When you get to the point where people are telling you that you are very friendly, you will have arrived. You'll still not be finished, but you will know more about creating and maintaining friendships. Think about what you've gained! You have new friends, more fun, and support when you need it. With a network like this you will live longer, be healthier, and avoid many retirement pitfalls, such as depression and loneliness.

Good friends are not born. Good friends are made, which takes practice and consistent effort. So, what can you do to keep up the momentum? Here are some ideas.

Idea 1: Repeat the steps

I mentioned earlier that you might be coming back to the venue list. Now is your opportunity. After you've followed the first set of SMART goals, go back and review the list. After your initial efforts and, maybe because of your initial efforts, you may have more information. A garden club may *not* meet at the community center.

Great. This information is still progress. You can cross that place off your list. But, keep going. Where else can you go to learn about gardening? Hmm. What about a home tour? Maybe if you visit homes with gardens, you'll find folks interested in gardening and can work at the effort from that end. Great. When is the next tour?

Get the idea? One step or one SMART goal may not complete the cycle in a way that works for you. Back up, turn the car a little, and pull out in a new direction. You'll get there. Don't give up. Remember the benefit list I just summarized: a network of fun and support.

I hate to nag, but it is true that the more leads you follow, the more sales you will make. That strategy has a positive side—you are developing a new "groove." As you begin to get the hang of it, reaching out gets easier.

Don't be discouraged. When you were younger, the first three play dates with Susie, you hit her over the head with your stuffed bear. Susie cried each time. But your parents knew a secret you had to learn: To make friends, you have to keep working at it. Eventually, you stopped hitting Susie and you've been friends ever since.

Friendship is a process. Or, maybe a better word is *organic*: Friendship is a growing thing. And like every other growing thing it needs time and attention. You can't give up feeding it or watering it or it will wither and fade away.

Do try to schedule regular maintenance. Maybe make it a SMART goal:

Every Tuesday I'll

- *Review my SMART goal results for the week*
- *Set some new goals*
- *Read another article on friendship*

It's not as though you have to get your graph paper out and chart a path. But you absolutely must devote time if your friendship network is to grow.

Idea 2: Journal your efforts

Your intentionality is at stake here. If you are serious about friendliness as an ongoing effort, you need a way to talk to yourself about how to move forward.

I'm not big on journals or diaries, but I totally understand about making notes on a software project. Keeping notes may be particularly helpful when you have a large nut to crack. It may take several iterations to arrive at a process that works efficiently. Unless you keep notes, you can easily cross back over the same avenues you've already tried that didn't work or didn't work well.

Think of the notes as the lab books you kept in science class or on the job. When you had a lab, you took notes about what worked and what didn't. What did you observe? What does that suggest? Do you have any more hypotheses?

Making or having a friend is not the same as having a lab rat, however. This approach is not nearly as clinical or as thorough. You are concerned about good results. You can use these notes to avoid duplication, note exceptions, and make suggestions.

Put your notes, papers with venues, activities, and SMART goals in a notebook, where it can help you see progress, movement, and change.

A notebook is also a place where you can put reminders. For example, the church you researched did not have a garden club as you thought it might, but the women's group hosts a garden party every April. Write a note to remind yourself of the event.

Reread your notebook every so often. The reading can give you an overview of where you've been and a possible new vantage point.

Idea 3: Be of service

I mentioned we value our Monday night dinners as a real bonding occasion with both family and friends. It is also a good place to make new friends as situations change. It reminds us to be invitational and inclusive.

But I didn't tell the whole story.

Long ago and faraway my wife went to graduate school. Sounds easy, right? Well, figuring out how to do that wasn't. We both had full-time jobs, we were raising a school-age daughter, and we were heavily invested in various activities. Going to graduate school smashed into that structure with new demands. I imagine you've had similar experiences and can relate.

I'm not sure whether it was my wife's idea or her Aunt Eleanor's, but that's when we came up with the idea for Monday night dinner. While Crys was in graduate school, we hosted the family at our house for dinner on Monday night. My wife's aunt prepared all the food and cleaned up!

Wow. One night a week we didn't have to cook or clean. And, we got to visit with family members in the area. One of our big concerns about the impact of graduate school had been the potential loss of that contact. As it turned out, the Monday night meal solved the problem. What a wonderful gift! Thank you, Aunt Eleanor.

As I mentioned earlier, the group has disbanded, regrouped, and transformed through the years. That transformation had one additional implication we didn't expect: We lost host families, and the number of cooks dwindled.

Our daughter and her husband both have active careers. They are raising our grandson and have busy lives outside of work, as well. As Crys and I talked about the changes, we realized that, except for the two of us, everybody else at the table has to work for a living, while also keeping up with life's other demands.

The tables have reversed, in a manner of speaking. We can now do something for family and friends that was done for us. We host Monday night dinners. My daughter and her family and our friends don't have to worry about one evening meal per week. Plus, we can pass along a meaningful tradition and strengthen our relationship with the next generations.

We're not obsessive about doing everything, all the time. Dave might bring his world famous pizza dough and all the trimmings so we can decorate our own pizzas. Ellen may donate a portion of veggies acquired through a local farmer's co-op. Tom might bring the makings and show off the culinary skills he acquired while in college in Rome. Clare and Amanda have shown up with pie in hand from time to time. Even Casey, the college sophomore, graced us with her first-ever-baked-all-on-her-own batch of cookies. But most of the time, we do it as Aunt Eleanor taught. We provide a service.

What service can you offer? Can you dovetail the needs of your family with the needs of friends and the skills you have?

Idea 4: Establish rituals

I love the smell of roast turkey on the holidays. To me, Thanksgiving is not about the turkey; it is about the smell. When I smell turkey, I'm instantly transported to every occasion where turkey was served—almost every Christmas and Thanksgiving since the first one I remember; I think I was six. And, seeing that I'm now a fully certified holder of a senior discount card at the movies, that has been awhile.

A single thread connects those events in my brain, making each holiday a more special occasion than it might have been by itself. The joy is compounded interest on an investment made over and over. That is the meaning of ritual: compounded interest on an investment—an investment in happiness.

The investment spills over too. The promise of Christmas or Thanksgiving coming is the prospect of another joyous occasion. Just anticipating the smell brings a smile.

Were all my Christmases absolutely joyous? Of course not! Top of that list was the one when my wife and I shared the Asian flu.

How about Thanksgivings? No. They didn't all make the trip either. My Mom refused to eat with us when my sister and I failed in our attempts to make the gravy darker. It turned out green. (In our defense, Mom did say, "I don't care what color it is. Quit fooling around and bring it to the table!" I guess Mom didn't like green. She left.)

But those exceptions did not spoil the occasion for me because the event was not one particular happening. It was a ritual that repeated itself. You can blow off an exception or two when you have a positive history of so many delightful memories.

Back in the little town in Ohio where I grew up, Christmas Eve was always a time for anticipating snow and caroling. One year when our daughter was very young, I talked my wife into going Christmas caroling. We've done it every year for over 30 years.

Here in Nashville, groups of carolers get together to raise money for a long-established children's daycare center. It's been a tradition for almost 100 years. So, when I started singing with a group from our church (that later became the band I've played with all these years), I invited them to bring their instruments and carol for Fannie Battle Day Home. The year it was ten below zero we did not take the instruments out but invited neighbors over instead. The ritual ties together the band members.

What is ritual? Ritual is doing things that are meaningful, repeatedly.

- Monday night dinner
- Serving turkey on Thanksgiving
- Inviting friends
- Doing special events such as caroling

Or, ritual is doing things until they *become* meaningful. We would certainly miss caroling if it suddenly went away. Invent some rituals with your friends and family.

One final hint for success: Remember the turkey smell? Our brains are wired to be sensitive to smell. Not all rituals have to be meals, but making a meal part of the ritual will have benefits.

Idea 5: Make your time together count

What did you realize you lost by leaving work? At work you

- Created something
- Built something
- Worked as a team

I've seen countless examples of what I call "meaning making" among retired people who are eager to give back. And, by so doing, they have found opportunities to create again, to build again, and to enjoy working with others.

- The band I've played with for 30 years conducts a gospel sing at three different nursing homes each month. The residents enjoy the music, and making music for them is a blessing for us.
- My wife volunteers at Saddle Up!, a therapeutic riding program for children with disabilities. My wife gets to hang out with horses and her horse-loving friends—two of her favorite things—and help the children.
- Our friend Larry goes to Florida for two months of the year. There, he works with friends at the mechanic shop next to their church, turning spare parts into three-wheeler cycles for persons in developing countries who have no legs.[19]

---

19 Check out The PET˚ Project sponsored by PET International. According to their website (petinernational.org), they've delivered over 36,000 vehicles in 95 countries.

- A retired minister we know spends hours on the slopes in Park City, Utah, teaching skiing. His students are blind or missing a limb.
- A retired seamstress we heard has made countless dresses for girls in an African village. She's now getting others involved in sewing—and serving.

Where will you reinvest yourself after retirement? You don't have to volunteer alone; you can take a friend and

- Build a house at Habitat for Humanity
- Help at a hospital
- Go caroling

Sharing experiences with others deepens friendships. That sharing becomes a new kind of "foxhole" experience.

You can also make your time together count by exercising. Talk about a foxhole! Nothing like a good sweat to build a bond, particularly when the rewards start rolling in. You really feel good toward a friend who has helped you gain strength, flexibility, and endurance; achievement is a great motivator as well.

Idea 6: Periodically review the situation

You have two evaluations to do every so often: quantity and quality. If you have never done this before, you might seek help. At the very least read some articles or books about friendship. The website for *Psychology Today* has a host of authoritative articles on a wide range of aspects of friendship. Take a look at some articles: (http://www.psychologytoday.com/basics/friends). What surprised you? What did you already know? What would you like to try?

What level of social network do you need? This is the quantity issue. Do you tend to be like my friend who could survive with a set of books in a cave? Or do you need a little more in the way of companionship?

What does your friend network look like now? Even though you may have lost friends due to retirement or attrition, you may not be totally bereft. You might actually list the names and places where you have friends now. Ask yourself the question about sufficiency. Frequently. Don't let attrition sneak up on you again.

You also need to address the quality issue with regard to particular connections. What can help this relationship? You can be too critical. Author Tom Rath suggests a "friendship audit," but reminds us:

> *It's not always a good idea to judge friends in a detached way, or to doubt a friendship just because you can't easily identify its rewards. The closest friends like each other for who they are in themselves, not for what they deliver.*[20]

But he does go on to characterize many different types of friends for the value they bring to your life. For example,

Champions stand up for you.
Companions are there for you.
Navigators give advice or direction.

This book, *Vital Friends*, is worth checking out just to heighten your sensitivity. Pay attention to the nuances these categories bring to your view of what your friends do.

And wouldn't it be interesting if you were to categorize the things you do for your friends? Do you fill the same role for each friend?

Blogger Laurie Pawlik-Klenlen suggests six ways to be a good friend:

---

20 *Vital Friends: The People You Can't Afford to Live Without*, by Tom Rath, Gallup Press: September 2006

- Spend quality time.
- Make friends your priority.
- Be there for the good and bad.
- Don't keep score.
- Notice the little things.
- Focus on the positive.[21]

Finally, you need to value younger friends. Writer Laura L. Carstensen suggests that you

Diversify your social network by befriending a person from a different generation.[22]

Younger friends can offer you so much:

- **Perspective**: Younger eyes bring a different viewpoint. We know how differences between generations can be the butt of jokes. My mother never saw the humor in saving the cotton balls at the top of a pill bottle from the pharmacy. After all, she remembered the frugalness of parents who lived through the Depression. Accepting the idea that saving those cotton balls might be less important, even humorous, is a step toward gaining perspective and a sign of growth. I don't feel I must laugh. On the other hand, I do want to understand how something might be funny to another.
- **Myth-busting**: "Teenagers these days are nothing but troublemakers." Every generation seems to discover the truth for itself. Never mind that you and your classmates may have taken great glee in tipping over the outhouse. At the time, did you even care that you and your ilk were nothing but troublemakers? Beware: The

<hr/>

21 "How to Be a Good Friend—6 Friendship Tips," by Laurie Pawlik-Kienlen, Psychology Suite 101, March 22, 2007. Copyright ©2007 Laurie Pawlik-Kienlen
22 "The Resolution of a Lifetime," by Laura L. Carstensen, *AARP Bulletin*, January/February, 2012

mind plays tricks on our beliefs. If we call a thing orange, we begin to smell fruit. We want to avoid saying things that are untrue for fear of believing things that are untrue.

- **Stimulating**: Do I walk out of the house texting my friends? No. But it is interesting to me to know why so many people do. How can I learn anything new if I'm unwilling to ask those questions? We're of an age where stimulating the brain is a guard against dementia. Talking with, being with, and trying to understand younger people from a different generation is good for me.
- **A Buffer**: Do you remember the nursing home? When your age creeps upward, the number of friends your age dwindles. Younger friends are a buffer against total loss.

And that is but a partial list of benefits of our having younger friends. But what is the benefit to them? If I reach out, I may give that generation some insight into aging. After all, they will learn something when they can go home and ask themselves why I did a particular thing or didn't laugh at an event they thought worthy. Stereotypes can be dispelled.

Another way to improve your friendship skills is to be mindful of the qualities you value in a friend. Take a look at the following list:

As a friend I

- Spend time with friends doing the things they want to do.
- Think of fun and interesting things to do with them.
- Influence my friends to do the right thing.
- Encourage them not to do things that would get them (or me) in trouble.

- Cheer them up when they are hurt, sad, or unhappy.
- Encourage and help them do their best.
- Am happy for my friends when they do well.
- Apologize when I have been hurtful, mean, or angry with them.
- Forgive them when they apologize to me. Make up quickly.
- Can be trusted to keep secrets they share with me.
- Tell them off (respectfully) when they deserve it.
- Am loyal—I don't talk about them behind their backs.
- Listen when my friends have something important to talk about.
- Stick up for my friends; don't allow other people to say mean things to or about them.
- Tell them the truth even when they might not like it.
- Find things we can do that are of service to others or the world.

I suggest you do several things with this list. **First,** make it your own. Take off the things on the list you don't value and add ones you do.

Second, test your friend-ability by giving yourself a rating for each item:

As a friend I

1. Seldom do this
2. Sometimes do this
3. Usually do this
4. Almost always do this

Add up your score—the higher it is, the better. Write the result and date in your journal. (See "Idea 2: Journal your efforts.") Add some reflections on the result and maybe some goals. Particularly note the things you'd like to improve.

Third, return to this list in a few months. Set a reminder on your calendar. When you review the list a subsequent time, complete the same process.

And then ask some new questions: What do I value now that I did not value before or vice versa? How did I do this time? Generally, your score should go up. Of course, if you are good already at these things or when you get good at these things, your progress may be less. That is a good thing.

Reviewing questionnaire results is not only about how good you are at certain things, but it is also about being conscious of the skills you need and taking the time to be reflective and purposeful about improving them. You don't want or need to show a 3% improvement over the previous year. What you need to do is have the intentionality and commitment to be good at the task of friendship. Numbers are not as important as good friends.

Idea 7: Don't put all your eggs in one basket

I think this bit of wisdom is important. One friend cannot be an end-all to your friendship needs or possibilities. This is true even if that one friend is a life partner.

If I waited for my wife to go to an action-adventure, bang-bang, shoot-em-up movie, I'd never see any. She doesn't much like playing pool either. On the other hand, if she waited for me before she went horseback riding, she would be stuck at home.

Last but not least, remember you don't have to share all things with each friend. You'll need a variety of friends—a network of fun and support—to touch all your highlights and interests.

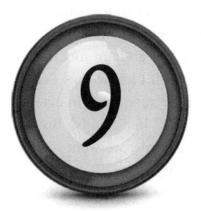

Love 'em

A word about families

I think the family is the ultimate "water cooler." It comes with the territory. You are born; you have a family. As a result, you spend a lot of time with them, particularly in your formative years. And, like the group at work, you meet challenges together:

- Going to school (Everybody gets to do multiplication tables!)
- Enduring puberty and all the changes
- Learning how to be a friend
- Growing in faith
- Landing a first job
- Experiencing a first romance

So, just like any other water cooler, you may or may not bond with the folks who drink there. I was not close to my family of origin. I was and am much closer to members of my wife's family. And, I know she is close to her family, as well. Crys and I have succeeded in extending this closeness to our daughter and her family. But that has happened intentionally. As parents, we went out of our way to grow the bond between us.

Just being a family member doesn't necessarily put you in the friendship category or transfer the ability to discuss certain topics. You build friendships with family members not because they are there, but because you've *chosen to invest* your time with them.

One thing to keep in mind with your children is that the relationship must change with time. While our young adult daughter struggled to not tell us everything as she had done as a child, she recognized the umbilical cord had disappeared at some point. Similarly, we realized she was perfectly capable of giving us a guided tour of her favorite haunts in England. We knew she had grown up. We are grateful to note she was and still is quite capable.

Would I rather have had a close relationship with my parents? Oh, yes. The lack was particularly telling in the last year of my mother's life. She refused to discuss nursing homes or other end-of-life options. Her emotions ran deep, and she was unwilling for me to bring them to the surface.

However, her reticence was pivotal to our concern that such issues be addressed in our family. I wanted my daughter and her husband to have conversations with us while we were still able to do so and not under the gun to make immediate decisions. Several months ago we finished completing the Five Wishes[23] form in dialogue with our daughter and son-in-law. This form deals with end-of-life issues including

- The person I want to make care decisions for me when I can't
- The level of medical treatment I want or don't want
- How comfortable I want to be
- How I want people to treat me
- What I want my loved ones to know

For my son-in-law the conversation was difficult. He was not used to dealing with these matters as a family. His parents, so far, have not done so with him.

In her last weeks, my mother decided all those concerns on her own. With her we had no advance discussion of the pros and cons and nuances that were a part of the end-of-life conversations in my family.

My wife and I are grateful our daughter has reciprocated our bonding attempts. Not because we can fill out a form, but because we have a high level of trust. At least, I think so. I hear periodically from her that I need to "behave." She says, "Remember. I get to pick your nursing home." Where does she get her sense of humor?

The few and the chosen

Most of what I've written about keeping friends or practicing skills applies to your entire network of friends, from the casual acquaintance to your closest and dearest. But you will

---

23 The **Five Wishes** document is produced by the Aging with Dignity program. The proper completion of this form meets legal requirements in 42 states as durable power of attorney and advanced directive; in the other eight states the form must be attached to the state's required form. See www.agingwithdignity.org

reserve a level of intimacy for only a few in your life. That level requires at least one additional step.

Some of your friendships move to intimacy, or love. I'm not talking about sexual intimacy—which seems to be the current limitation placed on the word. I'm also not talking about "luv," a puppy infatuation. I'm talking about a level of mutual caring and attention that surpasses the norm. I'm talking about bonding. I share that level with my spouse.[24] I characterize the move as a transformation from friendship to partner.

And for me, that transformation is marked by one big difference—I'm living with my intimate friend. Thus, we spend more time together. We talk more. We hang out more. We have more to lose if we blow it.

To get this level right, five factors are crucial:

- Being responsive
- Understanding your partner's method of showing love
- Overcoming barriers to good communication
- Turning tolerance into an art form
- Keeping at it, day after day

Being responsive

An intimate relationship will survive only if your partner perceives you are responsive to his or her needs. How do you do that?

Well, according to Mark Leary, a professor at Duke University,[25] you have to support and promote your partner's welfare. Successful supporting habits include

---

24 Maybe a couple of others can be that close as well. I'm not sure. I have close friends. Judging from the amount of effort I think I need in my marriage, I don't think I'd have the time for more. And, I'm not sure I'd be interested, either.

25 Lecture entitled "What Makes Relationships Succeed or Fail?" in a course called *Understanding the Mysteries of Human Behavior*, by Mark Leary, Ph.D., Duke University. Copyright © 2012; published by The Teaching Company.

- Providing help
- Endorsing the partner's goals and devoting support/time/resources to achieving them
- Paying attention to the partner
- Listening to the partner
- Celebrating accomplishments

Leary mentions the complications involved in efforts to be responsive. It isn't easy to be responsive. He says that the recipient is aware of these attentive activities only two-thirds of the time. Oops.

What does that mean? Let's use Crys and me as an example. I think I'm a fairly responsive guy. Sadly, of all the things I do intentionally to be responsive, Crys only picks up on two out of three of them (66%).

On the other hand, this pattern is saved somewhat by another research result. Apparently the partner claims being on the receiving end of attentive activities one-half of the time. So, Crys notices me being attentive even when I'm not trying.

Don't you just love freebies? You are halfway good at the practice of being responsive—without even trying. Remember what I said earlier: Friendship takes time and effort. But being responsive is only half the battle. You have to know what to be responsive to. What does the partner want?

Understanding love's variations

Gary Chapman has written an interesting book on love that delves into different ways people express it and expect it. He has identified five:

- **Quality time**: Watching a movie, taking long walks, and playing together are examples. Just being together will often suffice; we're not necessarily talking about deep soul-searching conversations every day.

- **Words of affirmation**: This style includes being attentive to what your partner does and acknowledging those things. In other words, show gratitude or praise or recognition. Say, "I love you."
- **Gifts**: Presents aren't just for birthdays any more. At least not for these folks. Of course individual taste may vary the level of expectation: Sometimes a box of chocolates will go a long way. For others the diamond necklace might jiggle the dial on the scale.
- **Acts of service**: Bringing water, tying shoes, rubbing feet are good examples. The bumper sticker, "Practice Random Acts of Kindness," could be the guidebook.
- **Physical touch**: Hugging, kissing, and holding hands are the craze here.

A mismatch between how we act and how our partner wants to be loved is a constant source of material for sitcom writers:

- **Wife expects hubby home for a quiet evening. Hubby substitutes flowers.** Things happen. I just had to work. What was I supposed to do? (Hint: Don't pass go; just head for the doghouse.)
- **Hubby expects an intimate, romantic dinner. Wife wants to paint the back room.** This mismatch used to happen to Crys and me. I think my wife solved the problem by starting an early warning system. Sometime in October she would say, "You know, when it starts getting cold in January, maybe we should paint the back room. Can't go out anyway. Right?" I've resolved that into every married man's year will come a certain volume of nesting duties. Sigh. She did give me plenty of notice.

- **Wife expects the garbage to go out and might want hubby to pick up after himself. Hubby is really good at telling her he loves her and she is beautiful.** Some people need to learn that taking the garbage out *is* telling your spouse you love her. Her complaint goes like this: "You say you love me, but I'd like you to show it once in awhile by taking the trash out. I can't feel beautiful if the house stinks."

In all of these cases nothing is wrong with either the expectation or the response. *But* the responses don't match well with the expectations. Have you ever heard the statement that it is as if the couple are speaking different languages. According to Chapman, this description is not an accident— it is exactly what is happening:

> *No matter how hard you try to express love in English, if your spouse understands only Chinese, you will never understand how to love each other.*[26]

Giving flowers can be a joke on a sitcom. On the other hand, it can be an expression of a man who values giving gifts as a primary act of love. For his spouse, missing the time together was the infraction. Flowers can't fill that expectation. The trick, of course, is finding out what your spouse desires. And, it probably wouldn't hurt if you knew what you had hoped for, as well.

Start by taking a look at how you relate to others you love. Say, for instance, do you find yourself doing things for your friends or giving compliments? High on your list would be acts of service or words of affirmation.

My wife's love expression is quality time. (I think. She also does affirmation well too.) You should see her with our

---

26 *The 5 Love Languages: The Secret to Love That Lasts*, by Gary D. Chapman. Copyright © 2010. Northfield Publishing. For more information, visit www.5lovelanguages.com.

grandson. She gets into the game, adventure, or build-it project of the day. She plays. She is present to him. I have a harder time with that.

You can also find out what your love language is by looking at complaints. If you're complaining you're not getting enough compliments or enough cuddles, your primary love languages are likely words of affirmation or physical touch.

Do you run into things at your house? I do. My wife opens the drawer of my desk to get a stamp. She leaves the drawer open and puts the stamps down on the nearest surface when she's done with them. I run into the drawer, of course. She puts clothes into the closet at bedtime and leaves the door open. I get up in the dark of the night to answer nature's call and run into the door.

What these observations say about me is that I value acts of service. I'd like my partner to close the closet door because doing so shows me she loves me. I'd like her to follow through with the stamp drawer because she cares about my kneecaps (not to mention my being able to find the stamps when I want them).

After 47 years of marriage, I've developed defenses to avoid severe damage to my body parts. Those mechanisms have not always been in place. It took me awhile to figure out what was going on and learn how to watch for open drawers after coming around a corner. Oh, I'm also less prone to getting upset about it these days.

> "Love is friendship that has caught fire. It is quiet understanding, mutual confidence, sharing and forgiving. It is loyalty through good and bad times. It settles for less than perfection and makes allowances for human weaknesses."
>
> —Ann Landers

I had not gotten her to change her stripes. I like doing for her. So I was disappointed that she didn't do the same things to show her love for me. I could never understand it. Isn't this how you show love? Chinese and English. Miles apart.

When you find out what makes you a happier camper, you can take steps to be happier. Step number one: Ask for what you want:

"I'd really like it if you would close the closet door," I say. I'm happy to report she's closing the door about 95% of the time now. Habits are important.

"Come play this game with us," she says. And thus, I'm enticed away from the computer (writing this book, maybe?) and on to spending time with wife and grandson. I'm learning to appreciate what my wife calls "a better balance" in life: a little work, a little exercise, a little play. It's good.

These examples lead us to the third means of identifying your love language: Ask yourself what is requested most often.

Chapman has another strategy for finding the love language you prefer:

> One husband told me that he discovered his love language by simply following the process of elimination... He asked himself, "If I had to give up one of the five, which one would I give up first?"[27]

Personally, I like Chapman's trial and error method. He suggests you concentrate on one language a week and watch the result. This appeals to the mad scientist in me. Pull the switch, Igor!

The one thing you don't want to do is take these discoveries for granted. Just when you think you have it figured out, something will change. Your primary love language may

27 *The 5 Love Languages: The Secret to Love That Lasts,* by Gary D. Chapman. Copyright © 2010. Northfield Publishing.

not slip away, but it may take a backseat at select points in your life.

Every once in a while, my wife gets into what I call her "project" mode. Usually this means she's got an editing assignment due soon. Often that entails putting other things, including me, aside for a bit. All this works out in the end. (Marital harmony hint: It usually works better when everybody knows about the deadline.)

What I've discovered during these periods of project concentration is that her primary focus of spending time switches to valuing acts of service more. In other words, guys: Your wife may need you to fix dinner, get groceries, and do other little things for her so she can keep focus.

One final way to find your love language is to do the exercise on Gary Chapman's *5 Love Languages* website (5lovelanguages.com). A different version is published in the book. Basically, the survey is a series of multiple-choice questions. Go for it.

Overcoming barriers

I learned from a business partner long ago that you just shouldn't sweat the small stuff. It has taken me decades to relegate some "I think these are absolutely critical, can't-live-with-any-exception rules for perfect behavior" to the dustbin. Well, maybe not the dustbin, but I've learned they're certainly less critical than keeping the relationship.

Is the "cherished notion" important to me? Yes. How about to her? Maybe not. I put this idea under the heading of fair is fair. If she is going to try to live with my quirks, foibles, and idiosyncrasies, I'm going to have to try to live with hers. That doesn't necessarily mean I think my values are any less important. It does mean that even though they are important to me, they do *not* have to be important to her.

On the other hand, you may end up doing things that honor your spouse's values that you may not hold. For example, I long ago gave up alcoholic beverages because my wife has a deep-seated, well-rehearsed passion against it. Abstinence has been her family's practice for at least three generations.

I was not unwilling to do so. My parent's marriage was damaged by drunkenness, and I was certainly not eager to see the mistake reenacted. But, at the same time, I don't feel the same way she does. I have a slightly higher tolerance. Even so, the marriage was more important to me.

In the early years of marriage, in particular, you run into the problem of discovery: *What do you mean you...?*

Ate that!
Read that!
Liked that!
Do that!
Continue that!
Believe that!
Didn't see that!

How many more do you need? These are the surprises of life—and the wellspring of marital discord.

Personally, I think you should give your partner a "gasp" quotient. You are allowed to "wonder out loud" the first time. After that, we discuss it.

The point being: Feelings come unbidden. What you do with the feelings is important to the relationship. It may take a while to arrive at the "live and let live" approach appropriate to the issue. And, you may not get it right. We all need some grace from time to time.

Turning tolerance into an art form

One of the biggest advantages to being tolerant is what I call the "do over," or allowing second chances. You can't communicate well all the time. You won't understand needs the first time every time. We all desire sometimes to be able or have permission to try again.

One of the single most important lessons here is to forgo consequences. In the real world, if you did that, the building would fall down on your head! In this world of tolerance, you don't walk away because you're slighted. You don't give up on your partner. You can stamp and shout. And, maybe you should. But, you come back to the issue and try it a different way.

I also think tolerance has a large laughter quotient. Just yesterday I bought chips to go with the dip my wife wanted to use for the caroling party. Only she wanted to use it with graham crackers. Now what dip do you suppose would go well with both chips and graham crackers? No dip that I know. Turns out she was talking about a sweet dip and I was thinking a savory.

The funny part: We've been talking about the dip for days and extolling its praises. We hadn't had it in a while. We were looking forward to it. And it was different from the one we made last year. All the statements were perfectly true—even though we were talking about two different dips.

We discovered the misunderstanding when I reached for the chip tray to serve our treat and she wanted a cracker tray. What would you do? We laughed. And we made the second dip the next day.

Practice tolerance. Laugh a lot. Your relationship will benefit.

Another resource you may want to look at is a book called *You Just Don't Understand,* by Deborah Tannen.[28] I did a workshop on this book some time back and remember one scenario I painted for the class:

> Judy decides not to buy a coat because it costs more than she and her husband agreed to pay when they talked about expenses. When she returned home she discovered that John had replaced the broken lawn mower with one costing twice the value of the coat she didn't buy. Judy did not know the mower was broken; they hadn't talked about it.

According to Tannen, men are socialized to be decisive. John decided that because the lawn mower was not overly expensive, they could afford it, and therefore he could buy it. Judy was socialized to value consensus.

Is it any wonder they had an argument? Tannen's book was a turning point for me personally because it pointed out some of the ways my training could get in the way of a relationship and how communication can go awry. As the training was really actually socialization, I was largely unaware it was happening. I certainly wasn't clued in to the kind of consequence shown by the example.

I couldn't tell you whether the same socialization process is at work today. But I am fairly confident it was at work years ago for most citizens of the United States of my generation, which probably includes many of you, my readers.

I've laid out several ways you can transform a friendship into a partnership or into an intimate relationship:

---

28 *You Just Don't Understand: Women and Men in Conversation,* by Deborah Tannen, Ph.D. Copyright © 1990. Published by HarperCollins.

- Being more attentive
- Understanding needs
- Practicing tolerance
- Uncovering hidden communication blocks

Some of these may seem similar to material in the chapter on keeping friends and also to the chapter on skills. I agree.

In other words, an intimate relationship is not a lot different from a relationship with our closest friends. The skill-set is similar.

If anything, the difference rests in how much attention is paid and how much time is spent. I'm with my intimate friend a lot more nights than I am with even my closest friends.

And, practically speaking, if I'm spending more time in the company of one person, it's more critical to get the needs, conflicts, and the communication issues worked out. I will have to live with—literally—the consequences.

Go back and look at the hierarchy of friendship diagram I presented early in Chapter 3: How many friends am I going to need? We discussed the fact that we might have numerous social contacts but only a few friends we could call our closest; the pyramid is broad at the bottom and narrow at the top.

The investment we make could also be shown as an upside-down pyramid. We invest little in casual contacts and much more in our close and closest friends. The pyramid would be broad at the top to represent heavy per-person time and energy, and narrow at the bottom representing minimal per-person investment.

Are there other things to look for with an intimate relationship? Probably. Go, seek out some more. Do I know them all? No, but I will keep trying.

Keeping at it, day after day

The trying part is what we agreed to the minute after I proposed. Crys told me I had to "try" two more times. Her family believed that a marriage decision was not a spur-of-the-moment thing. Consequently, I had to propose a second time and a third time. And she had to accept a second time and a third time.

Being intimate is a decision. Love is a decision. Both are commitments, made daily, and made even when you might not feel like it.

As a result of our commitment, Crys and I have undertaken various activities just to be married "better." We've read books, taken classes, and gone on retreats. We want to get good at marriage. So far, it is working.

I wish for you no less. Friendship is important. And a partner is a treasure of joy, companionship, and fulfillment. Work for it. It's worth it!

You want to know what I think about the "ask three times" proposal rule? I think she pretty much made that up on the spot, because she didn't know if I was joking when I said in a moment of passion, "I'll marry you, if you'll marry me." It's been 47 years now. Maybe this year I'll tell her.

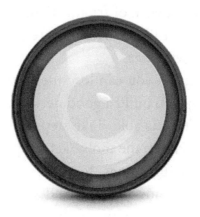

Conclusion

Retirement is full of surprises. One of the biggest is that you lose your friends.

How we cope with that can be a real challenge, based on how much we're willing to do to replace those things about work that made friendships possible. At the very least we have to

- **Devote regular effort** to growing our friendships
- **Be with people** where we can
- **Do meaningful things** together

The problem is not so much the immediate loss of certain acquaintances as what repeated losses mean for the future. If you don't work at making friends, the specter of loneliness lurks in the shadows. Timing is critical. During the early years of retirement, you have more time to invest in growing your network of friends than you did when you were working. You're likely to have more energy when newly retired than you will later.

As the years go by, you can lose the advantages you have now that can help you build a good network. You won't be as strong. You won't be as able. Take steps now to move in the right direction. Acquire the tools. Get the practice.

Doing meaningful things together provides a double benefit: You spend time together and you cement a shared commitment to the activity. If the meaningful activities include some kind of service, that's a bonus. The reaching out part will help you give back and will honor the gifts you've been given.

Belonging is equally important. It's not only about what you do for yourself that counts but also the companionship you have along the way. You can rebuild the "water cooler" on your own terms this time—a new place where you can make new friends. It becomes a reward in itself that provides blessings for you and for others.

This checkpoint is about trajectory. What course do you intend? Do you want to allow the loss of friends to continue until you find yourself alone? Or, do you step out and make the effort to set the course for being friendly and making friends?

You *can* grow your network of fun and support. You *can* have great friendships.

When you know where and how to find friends, meet them, and keep them, you have built armor against loss that literally shields you from loneliness and fills your days with interest and joy. You will be less likely to wait for folks to visit and more likely to be the one doing the visiting.

The trajectory also leads you to become the friendly person

that people will want to get to know and be with. The more friends you find, the more friends find you. The band I play with knew a lady who came regularly to our performances. At age 94, she would pop up and do the two-step. Men responded to her request for a partner! Go, girl!

And go, you! Get started now. Figure out ways to keep at it—and reap the rewards. You can do this! Do I see a two-step in your future?

More on SMART Goals

SMART goal components

Start with **Specific** objectives. "I will make friends" is a laudable objective but not a specific one. "I will meet Mike" is specific.

The specific objective in a SMART goal has to be **Measurable**. Putting a measurement to an objective helps you avoid vague or too broad goals that cannot be attained. If you can measure key elements, the goal is much more likely to be specific.

On the other hand, "I will make 5,000 cookies" may be specific and measurable, but that goal may be nearly unattainable, as well. You can overdo. Watch that the goals you write are **Attainable**.

Relevant is also important. You have to pick things that will make sense in context. "I will review three packets of pictures from my mother's ancient family collection this week." This example shows the beginning of an excellent SMART goal. But it is not relevant to the task at hand. Your SMART goals must maintain the focus on what achievements you envision. Writing those why or benefit statements might be helpful here, as well.

Finally, your SMART goal should be **Time-bound**. Setting deadlines is important for two reasons: motivation and focus. If I know I'm on a short leash, I'm less likely to wander around chasing the wrong thing.

SMART goal examples

The following list of SMART goals is categorized by type. This list was generated from participant input at the **New 3Rs of Retirement** workshops my wife and I conduct in the Nashville area.

#1 – Be a friend to have a friend.

- I want to be a good listener. My wife and I will be talking about summer plans tonight. Before then I'm going to review my active listening skills[40] and put them into practice tonight.
- In the meanwhile, this week I will take a vase of flowers from my garden to my neighbor.

#2 – Rediscover old friends.

- I wonder what my school buddy Peter is doing. By the weekend I'm going to search the Internet to find him.

---

40 http://www.mindtools.com/CommSkll/ActiveListening.htm

- Herb and Jeanne go from Kansas to Pennsylvania every summer. Perhaps we could meet them at a "halfway" point. I'll give them a call this weekend and see if they're interested.
- By Friday I will email my friend and arrange a lunch date for next week.

#3 – Find people with similar interests.

- Our church hosts a breakfast discussion group on Tuesdays. Next week I'll go check that out.
- I enjoyed discussing "meaty" topics in school. Maybe I can do that again. I think I'll call three folks this week to see if I can raise some interest in having a regular get-together for discussion on issues.
- This month I will attend the men's breakfast at church.

#4 – Invite someone to share an activity with you.

- John always liked science fiction too. Maybe it is time to check out the local club. I'll look up some options tonight, and invite him to come. *(Substitute woodworking, bicycle repair, football, black and white movies, disk golf, caving, archery, putt putt, for example.)*
- Haven't seen a baseball game in a while. A ballpark hotdog sure sounds good. Tonight I'll see if Frank and his kids would like to go to a game with me this weekend. *(Invite someone younger to participate in an activity that you enjoy too.)*

Other Books by Ed Zinkiewicz

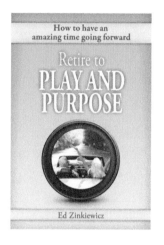

Retire to Play and Purpose
How to have an amazing time
going forward

Retire to a Better You
How to be *able* for the rest of
your life

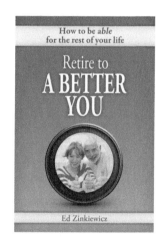

**Find more details about these
and other resources at**

Retire-To.com

CPSIA information can be obtained at www.ICGtesting.com
Printed in the USA
LVOW02s1102181113

361725LV00005B/8/P

9 780988 662261